SOMATIC EXERCISES
&
NERVOUS SYSTEM
REGULATION

Tools & Exercises To Reduce Anxiety,
Calm Your Nerves & Restore Mind-Body Balance

689 Burke Rd
Camberwell Victoria 3124
Australia

www.LearnWellBooks.com

We're led by God. Our business is also committed to supporting kids' charities. At the time of printing, we have donated well over $100,000 to enable mentoring services for underprivileged children. By choosing our books, you are helping children who desperately need it. Thank you.

This Is Really Important.
It's a Sincere Thank You.

My name is Wayne, the founder of LearnWell.

My Dad put a book in my hands when I was 13. It was written by Zig Ziglar and it changed the course of my life. Since then, it's been books that have helped me get over breakups, learn how to be a good friend, study the lives of good people and books have been the source of my persistence through some pretty challenging times.

My purpose is now to return the favor. To create books that might be the turning point in the lives of people around the world, just like they've been for me. It's enough to almost bring me to tears to think of you holding this book, seeking information and wisdom from something that I've helped to create. I'm moved in a way that I can't fully explain.

We're a small and 'beyond-enthusiastic' team here at LearnWell. We're writers, editors, researchers, designers, formatters (oh ... and a bookkeeper!) who take your decision to learn with us incredibly seriously. We consider it a privilege to be part of your learning journey. Thank you for allowing us to join you.

If there's anything we did really well, anything we messed up, or anything AT ALL that we could do better, would you please write to us and tell us (like, right now!) We would love to hear from you!

readers@learnwellbooks.com

We're sending you our thanks, our love and our very best wishes.

Wayne

and the team at LearnWell Books.

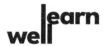

CONTENTS

BOOK 1

**SOMATIC EXERCISES FOR
NERVOUS SYSTEM REGULATION** 7

35 Beginner – Intermediate Techniques To Reduce Anxiety
& Tone Your Vagus Nerve In Under 10 Minutes A Day

WORKBOOK 1 133

BOOK 2

**TOOLS TO REGULATE YOUR
NERVOUS SYSTEM** 177

Somatic, Cognitive & Lifestyle Techniques
To Create Calm, Relieve Stress & Reduce Anxiety

WORKBOOK 2 297

BOOK 1

SOMATIC EXERCISES

FOR NERVOUS SYSTEM REGULATION

35 Beginner – Intermediate Techniques
To Reduce Anxiety & Tone Your Vagus Nerve In
Under 10 Minutes A Day

I wrote this for you.

You deserve to feel good.

BOOK 1 CONTENTS

Introduction   13

1   The Wisdom & Benefits Of Somatic Practices   15
     Creating Physical And Mental Well-Being
     Through The Power Of The Body-Mind Connection

2   Mastering Movement for Mind-Body Harmony   23
     Effective Techniques for Nervous System Harmony

3   Navigating Emotional Release
     Through Somatic Movement   30
     How To Recognize And Release Emotions
     To Build Emotional Resilience

4   Cultivating Deep Body Awareness   37
     Tuning Into Your Body's Language

5   35 Life-Changing Somatic Exercises   45
     Your Comprehensive Guide To Practices Proven To Work

     SECTION 1: REVITALIZING THROUGH BREATH   47
     Exercise 1: Diaphragmatic Breathing   48
     Exercise 2: Somatic Sighing   50
     Exercise 3: Somatic Breath Counting   52
     Exercise 4: Humming   54

SECTION 2: STRESS AND TENSION RELEASE   56

Exercise 5: Progressive Muscle Relaxation   57

Exercise 6: Body Scan Meditation   59

Exercise 7: Palm Pushing   61

Exercise 8: Leg Shaking   63

Exercise 9: Trauma-Releasing Exercises (Tre)   65

Exercise 10: Somatic Writing   67

Exercise 11: Guided Imagery   69

SECTION 3: SPINAL AND POSTURAL HEALTH   71

Exercise 12: Pelvic Tilts   72

Exercise 13: Spinal Twists   74

Exercise 14: Cat-Cow Stretch   76

Exercise 15: Rolling Down The Spine   78

Exercise 16: Child's Pose   80

Exercise 17: Seated Forward Bend   82

Exercise 18: Standing Forward Bend   84

SECTION 4: MINDFULNESS AND GROUNDING   86

Exercise 19: Grounding Exercises   87

Exercise 20: Mindful Walking   90

Exercise 21: Eye Palming   92

Exercise 22: Somatic Visualization   94

Exercise 23: Yoga Sun Salutations   96

SECTION 5: GRACEFUL MOVEMENTS FOR FLEXIBILITY   **99**

Exercise 24: Tai Chi Movements   100

Exercise 25: Butterfly Pose   102

Exercise 26: Cross-Crawl Exercise   104

Exercise 27: Arm Stretching And Releasing   106

Exercise 28: Side Bends   108

Exercise 29: Knee-To-Chest Stretch   110

Exercise 30: Figure-Eight Hip Movements   112

Exercise 31: Psoas Release Exercise   114

Exercise 32: Lateral Neck Stretch   116

Exercise 33: Self-Massage   118

SECTION 6: BALANCE AND FOCUS   **120**

Exercise 34: Balancing On One Foot   121

Exercise 35: Somatic Empathy Exercise   123

6   Your Personalized Somatic Exercise Plan   125
     10 Minutes Per Day For A Harmonized Nervous System

Conclusion   131

References   132

WORKBOOK

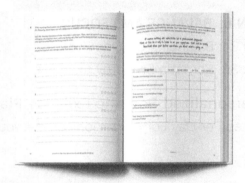

The average reader remembers just 14% of what they read. To increase the amount of knowledge you absorb on this important topic, we have included a user-friendly Workbook that follows the content of this book, chapter by chapter. You will find the Workbook located on page 133. Alternatively, you can download and print a separate copy of the Workbook by following the link below:

Download A Copy Of The Workbook Here:

www.learnwellbooks.com/embody

INTRODUCTION

The thought of therapy most likely brings to mind hours upon hours of talking where topics range from mundane to past trauma wound reopening.

The treatment for physical trauma is much the same – revisiting, medicating, and leaving the doctor's office feeling stuck with your burdens.

While many popular healing modalities have a purpose and a place, very few are able to approach trauma healing in a holistic, self-empowering way. A lot of chronic trauma sufferers, including those of us with chronic mental health ailments, have felt the powerlessness that comes from seeing doctors over and over again with little or sometimes no progress toward healing.

Before I learned about somatic exercise, I had already taken my healing into my own hands. However, upon facing mental health challenges that manifested in a very real and physical way, I was forced to try something new. I could no longer get away with intellectualizing my trauma. I had to stop and let myself feel.

Now, years after that unexpected hospital visit, somatics have changed my life. I have gained a sense of safety within my body that is becoming increasingly easy to return to after stress. All I can wish for is that sharing what I've learned can help change your life, too.

You don't need to be or see a professional somatic practitioner to experience big progress, either. The exercises in this book are some of the most widely used and effective somatic exercises, regardless of your experience level.

I've split the information into 6 simple chapters, 4 of which hold all the basic information you need on somatics to understand why it works and how you can get started. The final 2 chapters are all about the exercises, with Chapter 5 acting as a vault for the 35 somatic exercises you will learn. As for Chapter 6, this is where you create your own personalized 10-minute somatic exercise program that you can complete every day for life-changing results.

I'm so eager to share this information with you. Somatic practice is truly a breakthrough healing modality, proving just how important the mind-body connection is in both physical and mental trauma cases. However, even without trauma, somatic practice is a powerful tool in regulating emotions and building self-awareness. A nervous system in harmony can improve your life, regardless of your struggles.

Humans will never be void of stress. That's what our nervous systems were built to protect us from. But with modern lifestyles, our nervous systems have adapted to cope in a dysregulated state of chronic survival mode.

It doesn't have to be that way.

With a quick 10-minute daily somatic practice, we can train the nervous system to regulate and return to harmony after stress. If you're ready to learn a skill that will carry you through all of life's burdens in an empowering and productive way, keep reading. Join me in Chapter 1, where we will start this journey off at the deep end of all the incredible benefits of somatic practice.

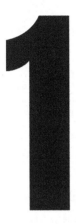

THE WISDOM & BENEFITS OF SOMATIC PRACTICES

Creating Physical And Mental Well-Being Through The Power Of The Body-Mind Connection

"There's no question that the mind-body connection is real, even if we can't quantify it. Hope is one of the greatest weapons we have to fight disease."

– David Agus

The gnawing feeling in my stomach had transformed into nausea, the slight imbalance in my stature became sways of rocking dizziness, and the spiraling thoughts in my head twisted into a slew of confusion as my body went into a shivering shock. I picked up the phone and called my partner for help. This was a medical emergency.

By the time he arrived, my legs had given way beneath me. The blurry reality around me blurred into blackness as I cried out, "I'm not ready to die!" I couldn't believe my life was over at the young age of 26. There was pain for a moment and then numbness. But things then took an unexpected turn.

I felt my partner's arms carrying me to the vehicle, and my blurry vision returned. The cool air of the air conditioner caressed my cheek as relief that I was still breathing washed over me. We arrived at the emergency department.

By the time a doctor came, I could walk, talk, and see normally. I insisted that there was something seriously wrong. However, multiple clear test results indicated that it was simply a severe panic attack.

This was beyond what I believed my mind was capable of.

Unfortunately, the panic attacks continued. But the cause of my panic seemed out of my mind's control. None of the techniques I'd known before seemed to work. It was as if the stress that I'd been under for some time had bundled up into a knot that continued to trigger my fight-or-flight response daily.

I couldn't escape it, trying to only made things worse. I had to accept and trust that this wasn't only a problem in my mind but in my body as well. So, after reading about a technique to soothe some nerve I'd never heard of before that was somehow connected to my fight-or-flight system, I decided to try it.

Knowing I would be alone for the next 15 minutes, I closed my eyes, sat up straight, and started humming. It was a deep hum that reverberated down my throat and across my chest. It didn't make any sense to me at the time how this simple exercise could actually do anything to help me, but I was so beaten down and lost that I was willing to try anything.

After releasing a deep, raw hum between each breath, I felt tears forming in the corners of my eyes. And then I laughed. A subtle sense of silliness washed over me, and the little touch of joy I felt was enough. I felt something other than numbness, worry, or panic, and I gripped onto it. If I could feel it for those few seconds after such an easy, seemingly silly exercise, then I could replicate that experience. "Maybe the joy could build, and I could feel like myself again," I thought.

It did.

After just a few months of expanding my efforts to understand and experience these exercises, I didn't just feel like my old self again. I felt better. I started to glow. The numbness transformed into a beautiful sensitivity and awareness. And on the days when I felt low or anxious, I could trust myself to work through those feelings and allow them. I made space for discomfort in my life, which inadvertently expanded into more inner safety, understanding, and joy. My digestive issues slowly resolved themselves, the daily vertigo I was experiencing subsided, and my physical energy levels improved significantly.

I didn't fully understand how or why these exercises worked, but my body didn't need me to understand. It simply needed me to allow it to *feel*. There were so many traumatic years in my life that I had worked through in my mind but never in my body. Every time I shoved an emotion down, smiled through the pain, and pretended I was fine, my body remembered. These exercises allowed me to sit quietly with my body and flip through the memories. They were all somatic exercises.

Almost any movement can be classified as a somatic exercise – even breathing. What defines it is the intention to release tension, stress, or trauma through movement. You naturally engage your mind-body connection when you use your body to release stress or trauma. This is the basis of somatic practice.

However, it's important to understand that bodies don't remember images or words as the mind does. It remembers physical sensations, emotions, and muscle tension. Taking the time to slowly release these "memories" through movement, breath, and other physical techniques allowed my body to lighten its traumatic load.

I'm excited to help deepen your understanding of somatic exercises because I know how effective they can be. I know how painful, confusing, and often scary it can be to feel chronically dysregulated. But I want you to know that becoming unstuck is possible. Somatic exercises are an easy addition to your healing journey that may very likely be the missing piece you've been waiting for – as they were for me.

For the rest of this chapter, I'd like to guide you through understanding these practices to further build your trust in them. I'll be touching on the interconnectedness of the mind and body, explaining the neurological systems these exercises work on, and how emotions impact the body. I will also unravel the importance of awareness for your mind-body relationship and what role that can play in an effective healing journey.

THE MIND-BODY CONNECTION

Your body and mind are intricately interconnected. It's difficult to affect the one without impacting the other in some way. When you are struggling with a physical illness or disease, the mind experiences changes, and vice versa. As a simple example, isn't it interesting how people with depression often feel physically fatigued or how low blood sugar can trigger anxiety? Our thoughts, emotions, and mental attitude can impact our physical health, and our physical health can influence how we feel.

In the same way, it's possible to heal physical symptoms with mental healing and mental symptoms with physical movement. The impact goes both ways. Somatic practices work with this mind-body connection to heal the mind by using the body while simultaneously improving physical health by releasing stored stress and trauma.

However, the mind-body connection is not a hypothetical concept. The mind and body are linked by a very important system of neuronal pathways known as the nervous system.

NEUROLOGICAL PATHWAYS

The human nervous system is the communication system that carries electrical signals between the body and the mind. It translates thoughts into actions and external stimuli into memory or mental experience. It comprises a complex system of neurons that spans the entire body and brain. That's why it has such a pivotal role in somatic practice. Regulating the nervous system is the core principle of somatics.

A regular somatic practice aims to improve our body awareness and muscle control to help encourage healthy communication between the body and the brain. It also aims to strengthen and balance the nervous system so that it can bounce back from stress quicker and with less negative impact on the body.

A nervous system that takes longer to regulate may produce uncomfortable fight-or-flight symptoms, inflammation, or other physiological changes for longer than necessary. However, a healthy one will allow faster recovery times if the body or the mind experiences significant stress or trauma. From sleep, movement, balance, and breathing to thoughts, emotions, perception, and neuroplasticity, the nervous system is connected to almost every aspect of well-being.[1]

With the branches of the nervous system connecting each of these bodily and mental processes, it makes sense that each of these processes can influence each other. One of the most impactful aspects of the mind-body connection is emotion. It is a powerful player within the healing game and is tightly woven into almost every aspect of life.

IMPACT OF EMOTIONS ON THE BODY

Emotions can have both a short-term and long-term impact on the body. In the short term, emotions often manifest various physical symptoms and sensations. Think about the last time you experienced conflict with someone and felt hurt or angry. How did your body feel?

Often, in these moments of heightened emotion, our nervous systems become activated, and symptoms such as a racing heart, increased body heat, sweating, and crying present themselves. It's also possible to experience an emotional shutdown, where we close ourselves off, suppress the emotions to avoid them, or protect ourselves from them, and other symptoms present themselves, such as numbness.

Suppressing or struggling to properly process big emotions can lead to a long-term emotional impact on the body. This is often when our bodies store these excess emotions in the form of tense muscles, weakened immune function, and chronic health issues. When we don't fully process emotions or trauma and instead carry them with us, it requires energy. Slowly, this extra weight of unprocessed baggage weighs our nervous systems down.

Think about a hot air balloon. Your body is the basket and balloon, while your mind is the passenger. The more you carry with you emotionally, the more you weigh the balloon down, making it harder to function. Somatic exercises can do two things: they can help you release emotions to lighten your load and enhance the working system of your balloon so it can function optimally. They don't just focus on one aspect of an interconnected system. They work to improve the entire system. And at the core of that system is awareness.

THE ROLE OF AWARENESS IN HEALING

By the time my chronic stress had triggered severe panic attacks, my nervous system was exhausted. I had ignored all the warning signs and continued to "push through," as many of us can relate to. It had become a habit to keep going despite the desperate internal calls to rest I was receiving from my nervous system.

Bouts of anxiety, derealization, nausea, vertigo, and more became symptoms I shrugged off and coped with to keep up with my jam-packed lifestyle and ignore the major stressors in my life at the time. Although I was an avid meditator before this point, I was too scared to sit still for a moment in my body and mind. I knew it would not be comfortable, so I avoided it.

In hindsight, while the panic attack caught me by surprise, there were warning signs for weeks, if not months before. My appetite had changed, I relied on daily intense exercise to take the edge off, I felt either tearful or numb on most days, and my evenings were filled with mindless social media scrolling or watching series I'd seen a hundred times before. I did little else to manage my stress because my time was limited, and I didn't believe there was much else I could do to change my circumstances at that point.

But there was one thing that could have turned things around much sooner: An awareness of my internal state.

The one thing I was avoiding most – feeling – was what would've, and eventually did, help me heal. Because emotions manifest themselves in bodily sensations, a sense of bodily awareness is paramount for addressing physical and mental discomfort.

Think about the last time you stubbed your toe. The pain lets you know that something in your body requires your attention and nurturing. Emotional pain is much the same. Think about the last time you had your heart broken or lost something important. How did it feel in your body? Did you feel a tinge of emotional pain?

An awareness of emotional pain and sensations allows you to identify where the emotion manifests in your body so you can better nurture and release it. Somatic exercises help to increase your mind-body awareness in this way.

ENHANCE MIND-BODY AWARENESS

Somatic exercises don't just accomplish one goal. While they work to engage and balance the nervous system, this can achieve many things. The intentional movements of somatics are designed to reshape neurological pathways in the nervous system to positively impact the mind-body connection. A strong mind-body connection can:

- Heighten your sensory perception
- Release muscle tension and stress

- Improve proprioception (sense of position) and balance
- Stabilize mood and thinking patterns
- Increase mindfulness and outlook

A strong mind-body connection is achieved through strong mind-body awareness. The more consistently you practice being in your body and paying attention to the sensations and experiences within it, the easier it is to notice positive and negative changes. Noticing the changes and working to release or process stress as quickly as possible allows your nervous system to move on quicker, reducing the time you experience the negative symptoms associated with stress.

Somatic exercises encourage you to slow down and spend time in your body. They ask you to become aware of certain areas in your body, sensations, and other changes or processes so you can release and shift them. Rather than speaking about a stressor, avoiding uncomfortable emotions, or trying to release stress in a way that might do more damage at times, somatics requires you to feel your way through healing in a manageable and empowering way.

I love the expression: choose your hard. Pushing away my stress and avoiding my inner experience with distraction, exercise, and emotional suppression made things feel less painful in the moment but caused more problems in the long term. However, slowing down, going inward, and feeling the pain I knew I was experiencing deep down was harder in the moment but made things easier in the long term.

Choosing to practice somatic exercises is choosing a little bit of potential discomfort regularly to reduce significant discomfort in the long term. However, the best part about them is that they can feel extremely healing while often being the most relaxing and centered part of your day. Like stretching a stiff muscle, somatics always comes with a positive reward, even if that reward is simply a softer brow, an extra smile, or a moment of harmony between your mind and your body. When you're ready, turn to Chapter 2 and prepare yourself for the practical aspects of somatics you need to know before attempting the exercises.

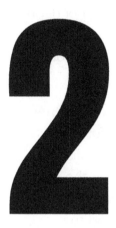

MASTERING MOVEMENT FOR MIND-BODY HARMONY

Effective Techniques for Nervous System Harmony

"Much ill health is due to emotional congestion. Constant rythmical movement is necessary to health and harmony."

– Emmet Fox

Growing up, I often felt a little rough around the edges. While I tried my best to have a calm demeanor, inside, I was either a bit jittery or completely numb. Finding a middle ground of safety seemed far-fetched. My nervous system was more often than not in some form of fight-or-flight response. My trauma still ruled my life.

As I matured into a young woman, determined to overcome her depression and anxiety, mindfulness, meditation, and other regulating practices became a part of my daily routine. Even without understanding the full neurological impact, my health improved significantly – but not all the way.

Although many things can regulate the nervous system, having an active understanding of how can make all the difference. As awful as the panic attack in my late 20s was, it led me on a path of nervous system discovery. Knowing how to safely explore the sensations in my body and my thoughts created a sense of harmony between them. Rather than panicking at the first sign of discomfort, I could sit with it, acknowledge it, and respond to it.

Nervous system harmony is not about never feeling dysregulated or uncomfortable. It's about feeling empowered to respond to dysregulation. It's about finding balance within both regulated and dysregulated states. Knowing how somatic movement influences these states will allow you to start from a place of empowerment and understanding to navigate the experience in the most healing way.

CORE PRINCIPLES OF SOMATIC MOVEMENT

Somatic movement is a tool for building awareness and a tool of response. It can and should be used for all states of the nervous system. The more readily you can engage in a somatic movement in times of stress, the more effective it will be. This comes from practicing even when everything feels normal or good. The awareness you build allows you to better identify your unique stress response and take action quickly.

There are several core principles supporting somatic movement, each one touching on a different area of the nervous system:

- Mind-body connection: Somatic movements integrate the mind and the body by promoting a heightened awareness of your bodily sensations and movements to better understand your body's unique response to stimuli, stress, or emotions.

- Breath awareness: Intentional breathing is a foundational skill in somatic practice. It helps switch your nervous system response from fight-or-flight to 'rest and digest,' promoting relaxation and well-being.

- Mindful movement: The core movements of a somatic practice involve slow, intentional movements that promote a sense of focus and relaxation while building bodily awareness.

- Tension release: Stress and trauma, both physical and mental, may cause chronic muscle tension. Somatic movement is designed to target and release this tension in a physically and emotionally healing way.

- Neuroplasticity: The brain is an organ that can continue to heal and grow throughout our lives. Mindful somatic movement can rewire neural pathways to build a more balanced and regulated nervous system.

Because the nervous system spans the entire body, somatic movement works holistically to heal and harmonize each area of the body and mind. For example, if you have a tight and painful shoulder, it can help to release the pain, tension, and stress related to the problem.

The key to using somatic movement in a way that works best for you is picking exercises that target the most dysregulated areas of your nervous system. Your body sends signals to communicate what it needs. Your mind needs to acknowledge those signals so that you can respond as quickly and effectively as possible.

RECOGNIZING BODY SIGNALS

The nervous system is an intricate web whose corners reach the top of our heads and the tips of our toes and fingers. When something goes wrong somewhere along the web, our body sends a signal to our brain. This signal is a message with a lot of information, but it is often coded in physical sensations such as pain, tingling, temperature change, or other bodily changes.

Because of our mind-body connection, even a mental change can stimulate our bodies. Our bodies are the communicator that signals our minds about what's wrong. For example, if you watch a horror movie and feel the hairs on your neck stand up, that could be a signal that you're scared. Or, if you're taking a walk and suddenly feel pain in your right ankle, it's a signal that your ankle is overworked.

Whichever way your body chooses to communicate an emotion or problem, its signals are there for your attention. It's up to you to use those signals and respond to the important ones. For example, if your ankle starts to hurt while you're on a walk, you can recognize that signal and decide to take a break. Or if you hear a strange sound outside and your hair rises, you can get up and lock your doors.

Your response to your bodily signals is meant to remedy the dysregulation. But it's difficult to regulate dysregulation when you don't know what caused it or what it means. That's where an improved mind-body connection and awareness are so useful.

When you engage in a somatic exercise, it's important to:

- Close your eyes where possible.

- Allow your awareness to scan through your body.

- Pay attention to the areas that catch your awareness.

- Identify what or how you feel in those areas.

- Acknowledge the sensation.

- Allow the sensation to exist while responding.

- Choose how you will respond in a way that soothes that sensation rather than trying to escape it.

In your Workbook, there is a space for you to try out this simple body scan exercise. When you're done, use a colored pen or marker to circle areas around the diagram where you felt a significant sensation. Draw a line to each area and make a note of how the sensation felt. Journal your experience and write down anything that stood out to you. Then, answer the questions for future reference.

Somatic movement and mind-body awareness allow you to recognize body signals with care and curiosity. When you can do this, it becomes easier to decode their meanings and respond in a restorative way. These movements are designed to release stress on their own, but your mind-body awareness allows you to adjust movements according to your unique needs.

GENTLE MOVEMENT FOR STRESS RELEASE

Somatic movements naturally release physical tension and reduce stress because of how they are practiced. Although they are often called exercises and involve careful intentional movement, they are not necessarily designed to increase your heart rate or strengthen your muscles.

Somatic movement is gentle.

Anyone can reap the benefits of this practice. They are intended to be slow, relaxing, and deliberate. They might incorporate gentle repetition of a single slow movement, holding specific body positions, intentionally softening muscles, or moving between positions in a slow and controlled way.

Taking the time each day to work through just 10 minutes of somatic movement can give your body and mind the intentional break they need to fully relax. These movements promote relaxation and effectively release physical tension by calming the nervous system.

A calm nervous system naturally reduces heart rate, blood pressure, muscle tension, and mental stress. It can safely enter the rest and digest state, where the mind-body connection can experience safety and relaxation. However, although these movements are designed to work regardless of your unique needs, you can modify any exercises to get the most out of them.

ADAPTIVE MOVEMENT STRATEGIES

You may suffer from a health condition or physical injury requiring you to modify your exercises. Rather than ruling great exercises out, you can adjust them to better fit your capabilities and needs.

Sometimes, only a modified exercise may improve your nervous system health by avoiding unnecessary strain on your body and better targeting problem areas. You can modify exercises by:

- Adjusting positions to maximize comfort and release.

- Reducing the range of motion the exercise asks for.

- Using supports or props like pillows, yoga blocks, or a chair.

- Progressing only when you're ready and able to.

- Taking additional time to rest in between movements.

- Modifying positions to accommodate physical conditions.

Examples of modified somatic exercises would include choosing to do an exercise from a seated position if standing is not comfortable, using a pillow to support your back during movements that require back stretches or lying down, only doing a movement halfway if the full range of motion is painful or not possible, taking your time to sit up slowly from a lying down position, and even changing or combining exercises to better suit your needs.

Somatic exercises are most effective when you work with your body to complete them. They are about listening to your body and knowing when you've reached your limit. Because these movements are designed to soften, stretch, and release tension in your muscles for nervous system harmony, it's important to understand your unique mental and physical needs.

Your body will have plenty of signals for you to identify and use to help you become more in tune with yourself. Remember to maintain awareness within your body before, during, and after somatic movements.

Building your mind-body awareness will allow you to recognize and respond to your needs quickly and effectively. This paves the way for nervous system balance and regulation as you learn not to ignore sensations but to see them for what they are: your body's communication system – its voice. Now that you understand the practical side of somatic exercises, please join me in Chapter 3, where we will explore the emotional impact of somatics.

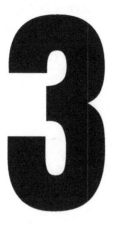

NAVIGATING EMOTIONAL RELEASE THROUGH SOMATIC MOVEMENT

How To Recognize And Release Emotions To Build Emotional Resilience

"The oak fought the wind and was broken, the willow bent when it must and survived."

– Robert Jordan

The floor seemed to push up against my back, holding me in a sweet, relaxing surrender. I felt at peace for a moment as the tension along my spine, hips, and shoulders melted into it. This was a peace I was able to feel on many occasions since starting a daily somatic practice, but what came next was new for me.

In that bubble of safety, something long-hidden emerged. It was a strange swell of emotion – neither good nor bad – that seemed to wash over my entire body. A gentle release of tears began, and I allowed it. I decided not to resist the experience and simply let it fully surface. The release became cathartic.

The emotions that surfaced seemed to have come from somewhere beyond the present, somewhere that was still holding onto what should have been released ages ago. And when it was over, I felt as if I could sleep. As the heaviness of the emotion washed away, a beautiful, serene lightness replaced it. I opened my eyes and felt moved for a moment.

Emotions can become "trapped" in our bodies when we don't know how to fully process and release them. Difficult emotions often arrive, even daily, for some. Imagine what that can feel like in the body when those powerful, heavy emotions stay with us. How does it feel to carry them around? The strain on our nervous system is major.

Emotional release is a big part of somatic practice. For our nervous system to become balanced, it needs to even the scales. If it's holding onto a lot of heavy, trapped emotions, it quite literally holds onto them by increasing muscle tension, inflammation, and more.

But when you release that bodily tension, the scales need to even out again. That's when the nervous system can let go of stored emotions. It can no longer carry them if it wants to stay balanced. The only way for it to release trapped emotions is through the mind-body connection. It needs to flow *through* you.

This is when somatic practice can feel daunting, but I'd like to demystify the experience for you. In this chapter, I will explain how and why emotions may come up and how to safely and successfully move through the experience.

Understanding the experience will allow you to deepen your practice without resistance.

UNDERSTANDING MOVEMENT-EMOTION CONNECTION

The mind-body connection allows the body and mind to have a bidirectional relationship. This allows physical movement to influence emotional states and emotional or mental states to influence the body.

For example, if you've ever been anxious while completing a task, consider how it affected your movement. Maybe you walked a little faster, became slightly clumsy, or spoke in a more jittery tone. Or maybe there was a time when you felt calm and rested. You might have moved more gracefully, had a lower tone of voice, and completed tasks at a more even pace.

The exciting thing about this bidirectional relationship is that you can use it to influence your physical and mental state. For example, when feeling anxious or jittery, you can use movement to release energy and stabilize the nervous system. In the same way, if you're feeling tense, you can work to relax the mind to relieve some of the tension.

Somatic exercises do both simultaneously.

A common problem that causes trapped emotion in people with trauma is a lack of safety within the body. Both physical and emotional trauma can result in this feeling. Pain can push us to detach from our bodies and emotions. Emotional trauma, depression, and anxiety can do the same. The more often we feel uncomfortable in our bodies and minds, the more likely we associate inner experience with unsafety. This is a big problem because we can't escape ourselves. But somatic exercises help us to feel safe within ourselves by creating small windows of safety every day.

Each time you practice a somatic exercise, the body releases endorphins, creating feelings of well-being and safety. The release of tension can feel relieving emotionally, and having a space to safely explore the discomfort of emotions is empowering. The more frequently we experience these positive feelings, the more wired our brains become for well-being.[2]

Over time, the moments of safety and well-being become longer and more of a natural state. This is because somatic movements influence our "feel-good" hormones and neurology. However, it's important to understand how to cope with uncomfortable emotions during a somatic exercise so you can safely recognize and release them.

RECOGNIZING AND RELEASING EMOTIONS

When resistance keeps you stuck, you can choose to release it to set yourself free. Emotions that surface during somatic practice are ready to be released. They might be uncomfortable, but they are only emotions. Recognizing when an emotion is trying to be released will help you see it for what it is, let go of resistance, and let the emotion move through you.

How To Recognize A Surfacing Emotion

Emotions manifest themselves in many physical symptoms and sensations. Recognizing when an emotion is surfacing will help you identify it so you can release it effectively. Somatic exercises are safe and gentle, so certain unexpected physical changes may often be trapped emotions coming to light. They may be subtle shifts, or they may be obvious. These symptoms and sensations can include:

- Physical sensations such as warmth, tingling, tightness, or tension.

- Breathing changes, such as breathing that becomes shallow, rapid, slower, or deeper.

- Facial expressions that reflect emotional states, such as smiling, frowning, or grimacing.

- Changes in heart rate, such as a racing heart or skipping a beat.

- Body movements such as trembling, shaking, or other spontaneous movements.

- Gut sensations such as butterflies, a knot in the stomach, nausea, or tightness.

- Mental shifts such as memories, flashbacks, or mood changes.

- Cathartic emotional releases such as laughing or crying.

- Vocalizations such as deep audible sighs, groaning, or other spontaneous vocalizations.

It's important to know that emotions may come up differently for everyone. You might experience a range of sensations, no additional sensations, or different sensations for different exercises. Getting to know how emotional release feels for you can help you understand when it's happening during an exercise. When you notice an emotion coming up, it's important to acknowledge it and release it if you're ready.

How To Release Emotions Safely

Releasing emotions can feel intense or scary if you're unsure what to expect or how to release them fully. If you suspect your body is trying to release trapped emotion during a somatic exercise, you can try the MY MOVE technique. It stands for:

- **M**indfulness: Practice being mindful of the emotion, acknowledging it fully.

- **Y**ield: Let the emotion exist in that moment. Don't resist it, yield to it.

- **M**ove: Use your body to move, shake, rock, wiggle, dance, or deep breathing to release.

- **O**pen: Keep your body language open to communicate safety and openness.

- **V**oice: Don't be afraid to make noises, cry, or laugh if it feels releasing.

- **E**ngage: Once the emotion has subsided, engage with your thoughts.

It's okay not to fully understand where the emotion is coming from. Take the time to immerse yourself in the experience without judgment and let the emotion flow through you. You can also take steps to set yourself up for success and feelings of safety by:

- Choosing a safe and quiet place to practice.

- Letting someone close to you know you're about to do a somatic practice.

- Using a journal to keep track of your progress and experiences.

- Reaching out for professional support to help you work through any difficult memories that have surfaced.

- Practicing your exercises with a liscenced somatic therapist if needed.

You can absolutely reap amazing results practicing somatics on your own if you are willing and able to release and work through the experiences. Somatic practice will help you build emotional resilience to better face difficult emotions in the present.

BUILDING EMOTIONAL RESILIENCE

The body-focused approach of somatic exercises strengthens your mind-body awareness so you can better recognize and release emotions. This can significantly build your emotional resilience.

Practicing these exercises regularly can decrease the tension in your body caused by long-term stress and trauma. But they also help to prevent the build-up of future tension as you learn to manage, regulate, and release emotions and stress as they arise.

The goal of somatic practice is to build a strong foundation of emotional resilience.

Emotional resilience is achieved through experience as you actively face and work through difficult emotions. This concept is a big part of somatic exercises. Emotions may take a while to come up and release once you start your practice, or you may start working through them immediately. Everyone has a unique relationship with their emotions. Somatics is about understanding how emotions come up for you and how you can release them best.

However, emotional resilience takes time and a consistent devotion to managing and regulating your emotions as best as possible. A somatic practice, even just 10 minutes per day, is enough to set you up for stability and safety from within so that you can confidently show up as your best and let stress move right through you.

A regulated nervous system balances both the body and mind. Emotions span between the two. When your emotions are allowed to flow safely through you, they no longer find places in your body to manifest for the long term. But it can be difficult to fully perceive your emotions and bodily sensations. What they mean or what they need to be released is also not always obvious

That's why cultivating a deep body awareness is vital to reap all the benefits of somatic exercises. When you're ready, make your way to the next chapter, where you will start tuning into your body and learning how to integrate your awareness into everyday life.

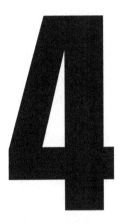

CULTIVATING DEEP BODY AWARENESS

Tuning Into Your Body's Language

"Attention to the human body brings healing and regeneration. Through awareness of the body we remember who we really are."

– Jack Kornfield

I had always been the calmest person in the room during a traumatic event. I could hold it together, take care of others, and do what needed to be done. In the moment, I would feel surprised by my amazing ability to cope with such hardships. And then I would crumble.

Turns out, while I was great at suppressing my emotions to get through a stressful situation, I had no idea how to manage those emotions when they eventually surfaced. They would bottle up inside of me until they'd overflow. Within hours, days, or longer, I'd unexpectedly explode with exhaustion, shock, and raw unprocessed emotion. It was either that or a deep, gnawing numbness. I struggled to escape the pattern because my emotions felt so foreign.

Everything changed when I allowed myself to slow down and *feel*.

Rather than bottling up the emotion just to get through the day, I started to make room for it. Rather than pushing through my chronic shoulder pain, I would allow myself regular breaks to acknowledge the pain and ease it. I started to prioritize well-being over being hyperproductive. My "on-the-go" nature was a symptom of survival mode.

Trauma has a way of overwhelming us. Although our instinct is often to pull back from the emotions and pain that arise, sometimes we have to lean in. Sometimes, it's better to listen a little closer so that we may understand our pain better. Becoming familiar with our pain and refusing to escape it is often the catalyst for its release.

Like a hand that grips tightly onto a balloon, our bodies hold onto trauma. By becoming attuned to our body's language and learning to speak it, we can give it permission to let go.

Being grounded in our bodies is incredibly empowering. Rather than allowing the mind to detach, weakening the mind-body connection, we can reconnect, touch base, and become fully present within ourselves using somatics. That's what this chapter is all about. I'd like to guide you through the process of enhancing your mind-body awareness so you can tune in to the unique signs of stress and relaxation your body presents, as well as how to integrate that awareness.

ENHANCING SENSORY PERCEPTION

Your sensory perception is like a muscle. When you withdraw from your emotions, ignore bodily sensations, and lose touch with yourself, your sensory perception weakens.

You might feel a well of anger pulse through your body and struggle to identify what you're feeling. You might rub arnica on your neck every night, wondering why it's always tight without understanding the core emotional cause. All your body's sensory signals feel blended. You hear the voice but can't make out the words.

Enhancing your sensory perception will allow you to tune into your body's signals to better identify your emotions and physical sensations. When you can hear what's being said, you can regulate and remedy the problems quicker and more efficiently. Well-processed pain and emotions don't need to stick around. They can deliver their message and move on.

To heighten awareness of bodily sensations, you can practice:

- Mindful breathing: Deep breathing exercises where you focus on the sensations of each inhale and exhale.

- Sensory awareness: Closing your eyes and touching different textures, taking your time to fully taste something, identifying different smells, or tuning into the sounds in your environment.

- Synchronized breath: Allowing your breath to synchronize to any physical activity such as yoga, jogging, walking, or dancing.

- Embodied mindfulness: Pulling your awareness fully into the present during everyday activities like doing the dishes, walking, or eating.

- Body scan exercise: A foundational sensory awareness exercise in somatic practice where you scan your awareness through each area of your body, noticing any sensations, tension, or relaxation you feel.

Like a muscle, practicing sensory awareness exercises will strengthen your ability to tune in and feel your bodily sensations. But it will also allow you to better understand them.

The more you feel and understand your sensations, the more patterns you will start to recognize, helping you make connections between sensations and emotional experiences. You'll start to differentiate between what sensations are there momentarily and which ones are physical cues with greater meaning.

STRESS AND RELAXATION RECOGNITION

Most involuntary bodily sensations hang in the balance between communicating stress or relaxation. Learning to understand your body's unique cues for either will allow you to feel in tune with yourself and navigate each state best.

When you can recognize your stress state kicking in early, you can take action to work through those thoughts and emotions before they progress to overwhelm. And when you can recognize signs of relaxation in your body and mind, you can identify what triggered the relaxation and take note of what's working. To help you identify patterns of relaxation or stress, here are some physical cues to look out for.

Physical Cues Of Stress

Beyond the mental impact of stress, some physical cues to indicate a stressed body or mind include:

- Muscle tension

- Headaches

- Fidgeting or nail-biting

- Fatigue

- Digestive problems

- Chest tightness

- Random aches and pains

- Rapid, shallow, or irregular breathing

- Unexplained increase or decrease in appetite

- Frowning or worried facial expression

- Increased heart rate or palpitations

- Struggling to fall or stay asleep

- Heat changes and unexplained sweating

- Dizziness or lightheadedness

- Poor immune function

- Closed off body posture

- Skin problems

- Grinding or clenching teeth

Of course, when identifying symptoms of stress, it's important to rule out other medical causes. However, when strange unexplained symptoms arise or reoccur unexpectedly, it's likely related to stress. Always see a doctor if you are concerned about a new symptom or experience worsening symptoms you suspect are related to stress.

Physical Cues Of Relaxation

Identifying states of relaxation can make them feel more rewarding and real as you consciously recognize the positive sensations. Some cues to look out for include:

- Soft, relaxed muscles

- Slow, deep and steady breathing

- Regular or slow heartbeat

- Improved digestion

- Normal, healthy appetite

- Falling asleep easily

- Feeling refreshed after sleep

- A sense of warmth and comfort

- Smiling or laughing easily

- Calm or happy facial expression

- Open, comfortable body posture

- Healthy immune function

- Improved chronic pain symptoms

Your perception of relaxation will be unique. For example, while one person may feel their body lighten during relaxation, others may feel their body growing heavier. The change will most likely be an improvement to how you felt before.

Everyone will experience a unique set of symptoms and sensations that indicate stress or relaxation. That's why it's important to determine what cues are normal for you. One of the most foundational practices in somatics is body scan practices as you have briefly experienced in Chapter 2.

BODY SCAN PRACTICES

The body scan practice is the foundation of all other somatic exercises. It is a step you should naturally include in each exercise you do from here on out. There is a full explanation and instructions for body scan practices in the next chapter. However, as the foundation of somatics, it requires some extra understanding.

During this exercise, you will close your eyes and mentally "scan" every area of your body, starting either at your toes or the top of your head. As you slowly scan your awareness through each area you will acknowledge any sensations without judgment and simultaneously breathe deeply and slowly. This process naturally indicates to your nervous system that you are safe, and it can enter the parasympathetic nervous system state, or the "rest and digest" state.

Body scan practices have long-term benefits on the nervous system as they strengthen your mind-body awareness significantly. They tune you into your nervous system and allow you to communicate with it. This is when pairing them with other exercises reaps incredible results. Providing you with that communication pathway, you can then use movement to further shift and release tension and trauma.

RESPONSIVE MOVEMENT

When you are fully tuned into your body during somatic practice it's easier to supplement or shift movements for the most benefit and release. This is called responsive movement. Because everyone is unique, responsive movement frees you up to adjust and move as necessary.

One form of responsive movement would involve accommodating your body's limits to help keep the exercises doable and comfortable. You could do any number of the adjustments mentioned in Chapter 2. However, responsive movement can also mean deepening the exercise in a way that feels releasing. For example adjusting the movement to target a certain area.

Tailoring somatic exercises to work better for you or adjusting them in the spur of the moment to accommodate new and shifting needs will deepen your practice significantly. While you will certainly feel a major difference with the exercises as they are, being flexible to change is what somatics are all about.

INTEGRATING AWARENESS INTO DAILY LIFE

Part of embracing the nervous system changes that come with somatic practice is allowing them to integrate into your everyday life. While a simple 10-minute per-day focused somatic practice is highly effective, you can deepen its impact by regularly tuning into your body throughout the day regardless of your emotional state. You can do things like:

- Pausing to take a few deep breaths

- Slowing down to savor a coffee or meal

- Grounding yourself during a conversation

- Replacing fidgeting with a short break

- Playing a song you love and dancing

- Smiling at yourself in the mirror

- Consciously easing your facial tension

- Taking stretch breaks throughout the day

- Focusing on sensations during menial tasks

Something as simple as tuning into the sensations of mundane tasks can have long-lasting positive effects on the nervous system. Tune into the coolness of the water when you wash your hands on a hot day or the roughness of a fresh towel off the line. Allow yourself the release of dancing freely around your living room to your favorite songs. Pay attention to the little signals of stress your body reveals throughout the day and remedy them with short breaks to breathe, stretch, or close your eyes. The little things add up the most.

Somatic practice is all about getting to know yourself. It's dedicating just 10 minutes a day to reconnect with your body and forge a deeper mind-body connection. It's listening to your body when you're stressed and leaning into relaxation. Learning to speak your body's language can change your life. To start planning your daily 10-minute somatic practice, turn the page to Chapter 5, where we will go through 35 truly life-changing somatic exercises. They're all simple, and anyone can do them. See you there!

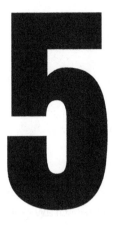

35 LIFE-CHANGING SOMATIC EXERCISES

Your Comprehensive Guide
To Practices Proven To Work

"When your body surrenders to movement, your soul remembers its dance."

– Gabrielle Roth

I hope you're as excited to learn these exercises as I am to share them with you. These 35 exercises are split into 6 groups, each with their own style and purpose. Some exercises are more geared towards stilling the mind and body, while others are there to shake you around and energize you. However, what they all have in common is their power and effectiveness. The sections include:

- Section 1: Revitalizing Through Breath

- Section 2: Stress And Tension Release

- Section 3: Spinal And Postural Health

- Section 4: Mindfulness And Grounding

- Section 5: Graceful Movements For Flexibility

- Section 6: Balance And Focus

As you read through the exercises, take note of which ones draw you in the most. That will be important in the final chapter of this book, where you will create your own 10-minute somatic exercise plan. When you're ready, dive into the exercises, and don't be afraid to try some of them out as you go. There will be space in your Workbook dedicated to journaling your experiences.

SECTION 1

REVITALIZING
THROUGH BREATH

EXERCISE 1: DIAPHRAGMATIC BREATHING

Diaphragmatic breathing is best known as deep belly breathing, an exercise that uses the breath to activate the parasympathetic nervous system. There is a vital nerve in the parasympathetic nervous system called the vagus nerve. The diaphragm, a large balloon-like organ that sits just below the ribs, is in close contact with this nerve, allowing deep diaphragmatic breathing to stimulate it and promote relaxation. This is a great exercise to start any somatic practice with.

Instructions

This exercise can be practiced sitting up, lying down, or standing. You can intentionally find a safe space to practice it, or you can simply practice while you're on the go, such as in the car, at your work desk, or anywhere you feel comfortable doing it.

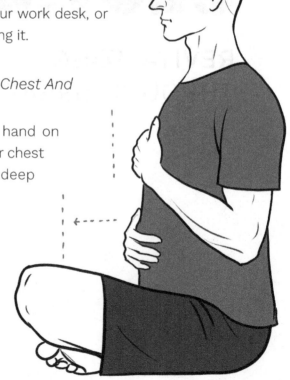

Step 1: Place One Hand On Your Chest And The Other On Your Stomach

In your chosen position, rest one hand on your stomach and the other on your chest to feel the rise and fall of each deep breath.

Step 2: Inhale Deeply And Slowly Through Your Nose

Slowly inhale through your nose, allowing the air to reach deep into your stomach. The aim is to see the hand on your stomach rise more than the one on your chest. This is how you know the air is pushing down on your diaphragm.

Step 3: Exhale Slowly Through Your Mouth

You can hold your breath in for a second or two before exhaling slowly through your mouth. Inhaling through your nose and exhaling through your mouth creates a nice rhythmic flow.

Step 4: Focus On The Rise And Fall Of Your Hands

Allow your attention to focus on the rise and fall of your hands, feeling the sensations of each breath both internally and externally.

Step 5: Repeat In A Slow Rhythmic Flow

Repeat this diaphragmatic breathing pattern for at least 5-10 breaths, making sure to keep a slow and rhythmic pace. Notice any shifts in your body and mind.

EXERCISE 2: SOMATIC SIGHING

Sighs have physiological, neurobiological, and psychological benefits.[3] They are essential for regulating our bodies and minds. Intentional somatic sighing is a way to use the function of a sigh to help us experience the benefits of sighing on purpose. A somatic sigh is an audible sigh used to release emotion or tension. It activates the parasympathetic nervous system, promoting relaxation.

Instructions

The somatic sigh is best practiced standing or sitting down with your spine straight and your shoulders square. Find a place where you can feel comfortable making audible sighs without holding back.

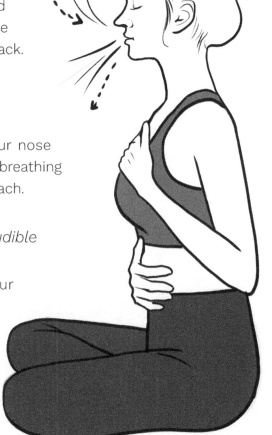

Step 1: Inhale Deeply Through Your Nose

Take a long, deep inhale through your nose as you would during a diaphragmatic breathing exercise. Feel the breath fill your stomach.

Step 2: Release The Breath In An Audible Sigh

Allow the breath to flood out of your mouth in an audible sighing sound. Release the full exhale as you notice any tension melt away.

Step 4: Become Mindful Of The Sensations That Arise

After each sigh, notice any changes or sensations you experience. Let those sensations help govern the continuation of the exercise.

Step 3: Repeat As Needed

You can repeat the audible sigh as many times as you like or until you experience a sense of relaxation. 1-5 somatic sighs are generally enough to experience a shift. You can also take a couple of normal breaths in between each somatic sigh.

EXERCISE 3: SOMATIC BREATH COUNTING

Focusing our attention on our breathing is naturally a great way to distract ourselves from pain or anxiety, but also to center the mind and improve mental clarity. To enhance the therapeutic impact of focusing on the breath, we can combine it with counting in a rhythmic fashion. Somatic breath counting is an excellent grounding practice for stilling busy thoughts and promoting a sense of calm. It is a mindfulness breathing practice.

Instructions

Somatic breath counting can be practiced in any position. You can complete the exercise anywhere at any time, even with others around. It also serves as an excellent regulation strategy for heightened emotions.

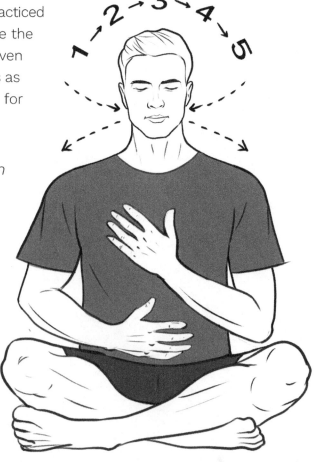

Step 1: Focus Your Attention On Your Normal Breathing

Bring your awareness to your breath, allowing yourself to breathe as normal for a moment. Pay attention to the natural rhythmic flow of your breath.

Step 2: Start Counting Each Inhale And Exhale

As you begin counting, start with 1 on your inhale and 2

on your exhale. Continue until you reach number 5. So inhale, 1, exhale, 2, inhale, 3, exhale, 4, inhale 5.

Step 3: Create A Continuous Loop

Because you ended at 5 on an inhale, your next exhale will be 1, creating a continuous loop. Simply continue to count from 1-5 regardless of which numbers fall on an inhale or exhale.

Step 4: Maintain Your Awareness

You may feel your mind start to lose focus from time to time. If this happens, gently refocus your awareness onto your breath, synchronizing your counting from 1 again.

Step 5: Experiment With The Length Of The Exercise

Although this exercise can work rapidly, you can reap more benefits by practicing it for longer. Set a timer for 1-5 minutes and experiment with how long you can maintain your focus. Challenge yourself! This exercise can promote better focus and mental clarity long after it's over.

EXERCISE 4: HUMMING

Humming is one of the most highly effective, commonly used, and ancient somatic practices. As the first somatic exercise I ever consciously tried, I'm excited to tell you why. Just as diaphragmatic breathing can directly stimulate the vagus nerve, so can humming. Humming reverberates through the vocal chords which are close to the most exposed area of the vagus nerve, the parts that run along either side of our neck. This stimulation triggers the activation of our parasympathetic nervous system, enabling relaxation.

Instructions

Find a comfortable place to sit, stand, or lie down. It's advisable to have some privacy or be with people you feel safe and comfortable around. While you can hum gently, it's truly great to be able to fully release during this exercise.

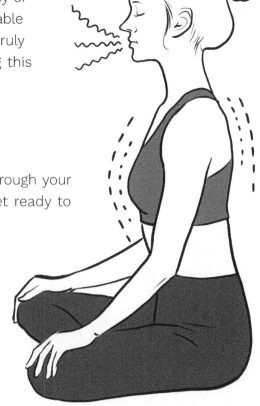

Step 1: Inhale Deeply Through Your Nose

Take a deep diaphragmatic breath in through your nose, feeling your belly expand, and get ready to release it in a hum.

Step 2: Release The Breath In A Hum

On the exhale, keep your lips closed and make a humming sound. Let the vibrations reverberate through your head, throat, and chest.

Step 3: Tune Into The Sensations

As the vibrations spread through your body, focus on where you feel them most, how they feel, and notice any relaxation cues you experience.

Step 4: Experiment With The Pitch

Play around with the pitch of your humming. Try a deep hum and see how far down your chest you can feel the vibrations. Try a higher-pitched hum and notice the areas of your face in which you experience the most vibration. Find pitches that you feel bring on the most relaxation.

Step 5: Bring Your Awareness To How You Feel

After a few breaths of humming, tune into your body and mind. Notice how you feel and pay attention to any shifts you experience.

SECTION 2

STRESS AND
TENSION RELEASE

EXERCISE 5: PROGRESSIVE MUSCLE RELAXATION

Also known as PMR, progressive muscle relaxation is designed to create awareness of any physical muscle tension you may be holding onto as well as offer a way to release it. Tensing muscles to release tension may seem contradictory, but systematically contracting and relaxing muscles can help release chronic muscle tension, build an awareness of muscle groups, manage stress, and promote relaxation.

Instructions

This exercise is best practiced lying down or sitting in a comfortable position. Choose somewhere quiet and private to practice this exercise. It's also advised to start this exercise by centering yourself with a few deep breaths.

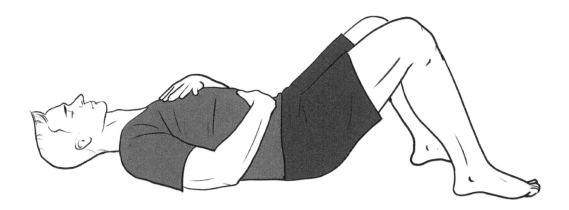

Step 1: Start At Your Feet

Once you are centered and comfortable, bring your awareness to your feet and contract the muscles as much as you can comfortably squeeze. Feel your toes curl and your arch pull inward.

Step 2: Hold For 5-10 Seconds

Hold the tension in your feet for up to about 10 seconds and get ready to release.

Step 3: Release The Tension Fully

Suddenly release the tension completely and bring your awareness to the sensations of relaxation moving through the muscles.

Step 4: Repeat On Each Muscle Group

From your feet, progressively move up your body, tensing and releasing one muscle group at a time. Tense and release your lower legs, then your upper legs. Move up towards your buttocks, pelvis, and hips, then your abs and lower back. Tense and release your chest, then your arms and hands, then your neck, and end with your face.

Step 5: Focus On The Contrast

As you move up your body, and after you're all done, take a moment to notice the contrast between tension and relaxation across all muscle groups. Notice any shifts within your body both mentally and physically.

EXERCISE 6: BODY SCAN MEDITATION

As we've briefly covered before, the body scan somatic exercise, also known as the body scan meditation, is one of the foundational somatic practices for increasing mind-body awareness and tension release. As you scan your awareness throughout your body, your perception of those areas naturally heightens, revealing insights into your sensory and psychological experience. A strong mind-body connection empowers you to tune into your body for information that can lead to better releases and relaxation.

Instructions

You can complete this exercise in any position you'd like, but lying down with legs straight and arms at either side may be the most impactful. This position leaves less room for your environment to interfere with your sensory perception.

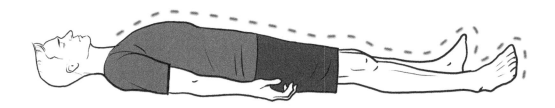

Step 1: Focus On Your Breathing

Start this exercise by bringing your awareness to your breathing and slowing your breath to a nice, even rhythm for a relaxing start.

Step 2: Start Your Scan At Your Toes

Bring your awareness to your toes and focus there for a second, taking note of any sensations or tension in the area.

Step 3: Scan Your Body Systematically

From your toes, move your awareness up your legs and through your body, taking a moment to mentally "scan" and perceive each area. Notice any sensations or tension along the way. Sensations you can bring your awareness to include warmth, coolness, softness, or tension.

Step 4: Release The Tension You Find

If you find areas of tension, focus your awareness on them for a moment and invite the tension to ease up. Consciously soften the muscle and imagine it melting into the floor.

Step 5: Move On Without Judgement And Recenter

Remember to stay mindful throughout this practice. Don't judge a sensation or resist it. Simply bring your awareness to it and be prepared to release it. When you've scanned your entire body, recenter your awareness.

EXERCISE 7: PALM PUSHING

Palm pushing is a somatic exercise that you can use to target tension release in the upper body. The exercise allows you to release specified tension by tensing and releasing the full set of upper body muscles. It's an exercise that can help with chronic tension in areas such as the shoulders, arms, upper back, and hands.

Instructions

This exercise is best practiced sitting up straight. Find a comfortable seated position in a quiet, private area. Take a few deep breaths before starting, and be sure to keep a regular breathing pattern throughout.

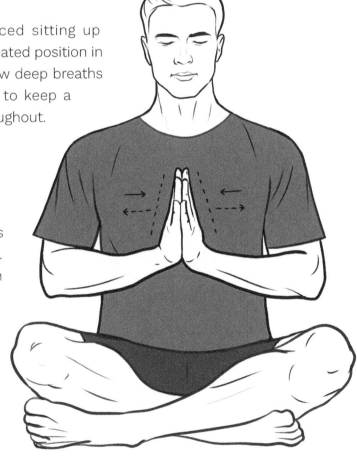

Step 1: Bring Your Hands Together With Palms Touching

Lift your hands with palms touching in a prayer position. Hold them together lightly in front of your chest.

Step 2: Push Your Palms Together With A Gentle Pressure

Now apply pressure between your palms, pushing them together with a gentle but firm force. Allow all your upper body muscles to engage and tense.

Step 3: Hold For A Few Seconds

Maintain the pressure between your palms for a few seconds. Keep the pressure comfortable and even make sure not to strain.

Step 4: Gradually Release The Tension

Keeping your palms together, slowly and gradually release the pressure and feel the tension release from each muscle in your upper body.

Step 5: Repeat As Needed

Continue to reapply and release the pressure between your palms as needed, paying attention to the contrast between the two states.

EXERCISE 8: LEG SHAKING

Neurogenic tremors are our body's natural regulating response to stress and trauma. We can see it in full action amongst wild animals, where an animal nearly escapes harm, and within seconds of being in safety, it shakes its body. Humans have this same mechanism that we have been conditioned to suppress to maintain appearances. However, this regulatory response is vital to releasing tension and trauma. Thankfully, we can simulate it for the same benefits with this leg-shaking somatic exercise.

Instructions

Find a comfortable place to sit or lie down where you won't be disturbed. Along with the incredible physical release you may experience, be prepared for any potential emotions to come up as well.

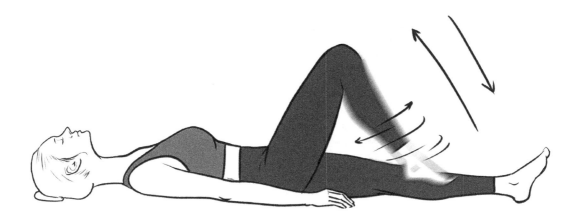

Step 1: Start With One Leg At A Time

If you're lying down, keep your knees slightly bent as you begin. Start with one leg, lifting it a couple of centimeters off the ground and shaking it vigorously. Allow the shaking to fully extend up your leg, freely and loosely.

Step 2: Tune Into The Sensations As You Shake

Continue to shake your leg for about 20-30 seconds, tuning into the sensations and vibrations you feel. Allow the shaking to loosen up any tension you may have. If you feel an emotion come up, use the intensity of the shaking to release it.

Step 3: Switch Legs And Repeat

Fully relax your legs again and switch. Lift the next leg and repeat steps 1 and 2, vigorously shaking and tuning into the sensations. After 20-30 seconds, relax both legs again.

Step 4: Try Shaking Both Legs For An Optional Full Body Experience

If you're comfortable giving it a try, progress the exercise to achieve a full body shaking by lifting and shaking both legs simultaneously. Allow the shaking to vibrate up the entire body and release stored tension and trauma throughout. Continue for 20-30 seconds.

Step 5: Reconnect With Stillness

After the shaking, sit or lie in stillness for a moment. Bring your awareness to the sensations you feel after shaking. Notice the contrast between the intensity of shaking and the sudden stillness. Take a deep breath in and exhale.

EXERCISE 9: TRAUMA-RELEASING EXERCISES (TRE)

These exercises, known as Trauma-Releasing Exercises, or TRE, are a set of lower body movements designed to fatigue muscles in a way that naturally induces the body's shaking or tremoring mechanism. There are 7 short exercises developed by Dr. David Berceli, which you complete in sequence to unlock stored trauma and tension.

Instructions

We're going to work with 4 of the standing TRE exercises plus the final floor sequence. Keep your breathing deep and flowing throughout. Once your body begins to tremor, let it flow for as long as you'd like. You can stop the tremoring at any time by simply changing your position.

Exercise 1: Heel Lift Calf Raises

Standing with your weight balanced on your right foot, using your left foot for gentle balance, complete about a minute of calf raises or until your muscle fatigue is at a 7/10. Repeat on the left leg.

Exercise 2: Hip Sits For Hips And Thighs

Stand with your weight balanced on your right foot, using your left leg to stay stable. Then continuously bend your right knee in a sitting motion until a 7/10 fatigue. Repeat on the left leg.

Exercise 3: Foreward Fold Stretch

Stand with your feet past hip-width apart. Fold forward and let your fingers hang to the floor. Gently walk your fingers from your right leg to your left, pausing at each to hold and breath.

Exercise 4: Wall Sit

Rest your back against a solid wall with your legs in a seated position. You should be able to see the tops of your feet to make the exercise feel easier. Hold this position until you reach a 7/10 muscle fatigue or start to tremor lightly. You can allow the tremor if you're comfortable.

Exercise 5: Floor Sequence

When you're ready, move onto the floor and lie flat on your back with your knees raised and feet on the ground. Slowly drop your knees into a butterfly position and rest here for a moment. Then, slowly pull your knees together, leaving a couple of inches of space between them and hold. Alternate between these two rested positions, allowing any tremors that happen to flow through you. If at any point you feel you'd like the tremors to stop, simply straighten your legs and rest.

EXERCISE 10: SOMATIC WRITING

Somatic writing is an excellent way to release emotions and stress by expressing yourself across the pages of a journal. Part of somatic release is releasing what is in your mind, especially when it's in a way that you can see and reflect on easily, such as with writing or painting. It is a great exercise for increasing emotional awareness, self-reflection, and stress release.

Instructions

Sit comfortably with a journal and a pen in a place where you won't be disturbed. Be prepared to write without a filter, even if you have to dispose of the paper afterward. If you can keep your journals private, it's a great practice to keep them for future reflection. However, many people like to burn or shred their journal pages.

Step 1: Set An Intention

Before you start writing, take a moment to acknowledge the emotions you feel or your mental state. Decide on an intention for your journaling that you feel most called to in this moment, such as releasing thoughts and emotions or gaining clarity and insights.

Step 2: Start Writing Freely

Without judgment or thought, allow the writing to flow freely onto the paper. Let your stream of consciousness

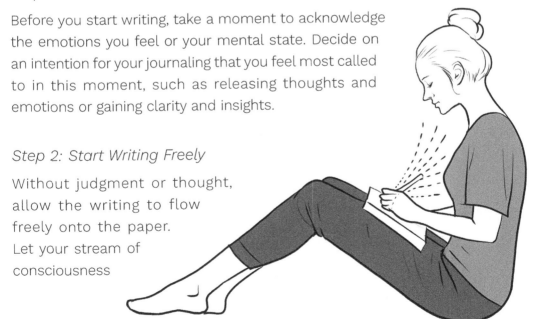

be expressed without censorship. It doesn't matter if the writing is neat or makes much sense. Be detailed and descriptive when addressing how you feel.

Step 3: Bring Your Awareness To Your Body

As you write, take a mental note of any physical changes or sensations you may experience. Notice any somatic experiences such as tension, softness, warmth, trembling, or any of the cues you learned in Chapter 4. See them as a release so your stress can move on.

Step 4: Reflect And Integrate

Once you feel done and ready take a few deep breaths. Take a moment to sit with what you wrote, reading it through and reflecting on it. Allow the insights to integrate by acknowledging your emotions and thoughts. Try to validate how you feel and refrain from judgment.

Step 5: Repeat Regularly

For somatic writing to be the most effective, try to implement it in your daily routine when you usually feel the most stress, such as after a long day. However, it's a great tool for emotional regulation for those times when your thoughts and emotions feel intense and out of control.

EXERCISE 11: GUIDED IMAGERY

The mind is a powerful thing that often can't differentiate between imagined scenarios and real life. Guided imagery is a way to train your brain into the parasympathetic nervous system state simply by vividly imagining you are in a safe and relaxing environment. It is a form of guided meditation.

Instructions

Find a comfortable place to sit or lie down where you won't be disturbed. You can either choose to follow a recorded guided visualization or you can proceed to self-guide the imagery.

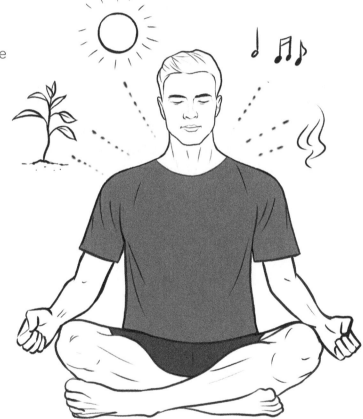

Step 1: Take A Few Deep Breaths

Center yourself and prepare for relaxation with a few deep diaphragmatic breaths.

Step 2: Decide On An Imagined Location To Visit

Think about a place you would like to relax in, such as a beachfront, a forest, a fantasy location, or wherever you'd like. This could also be a relaxing scenario like receiving a massage, going on a train ride, or whatever scenario you feel is relaxing.

Step 3: Close Your Eyes And Begin Visualizing

With your eyes closed, walk yourself through the visualization. Imagine all the various details of the location or situation.

Step 4: Engage Your Senses

Let your senses come to life within the visualization. Visualize the smells, the colors and objects you can see, the things you can touch, and the noises you can hear. For example, you can feel the cool water of a forest stream, listen to the seagulls at the beach, or feel the warmth of hot massage stones being placed on your back. Try to be as present as possible in your visualization.

Step 5: Complete The Exercise With A Body Scan

While in this fictional location, complete a body scan, bringing your awareness from your toes to your head. Notice any changes you feel and acknowledge them. Before you open your eyes, feel the visualization drifting away as you slowly move your physical body again. Finish with a few deep breaths and notice any relaxation cues you feel.

SECTION 3

SPINAL AND POSTURAL HEALTH

EXERCISE 12: PELVIC TILTS

A fantastic somatic practice for relieving lower back pain and tension is the pelvic tilt. The rocking motion of the pelvis helps to loosen up the muscles in the lower back and pelvis, releasing stored tension and promoting flexibility. Practicing regular pelvic tilts can contribute to improved lower back health.

Instructions

Find a comfortable place to lie flat on your back. Relax your upper body and neck fully with your knees bent and feet flat on the ground. Your feet should be hip-width apart.

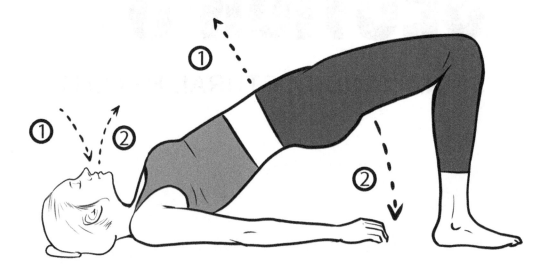

Step 1: Start By Engaging Your Core Muscles

Your core muscles will provide you with the stability to complete this exercise. Simply engage them enough to assist you without the tension influencing your steady breathing.

Step 2: Tilt Your Pelvis Forward

With steady control, tilt your pelvis forward so your tailbone moves further beneath you. This should create a deeper arch in your lower back.

Step 3: Release The Pelvic Tilt And Deepen

Relax your pelvis, allowing your lower back to return to a neutral position. Now deepen this pelvic release by pushing your lower back into the ground so your tailbone lifts further up

Step 4: Create A Rocking Motion By Repeating Steps 2 & 3

Continue to tilt your pelvis back and forth in a gentle, controlled rocking motion. Let the floor massage the muscles in this area, and the controlled movements tighten and loosen them to release tension.

Step 5: Sync Your Breath With The Movement

Take a moment to sync your breathing to the pelvic tilt. Inhale on the forward tilt, and exhale as you release and deepen. Repeat for a minute or 2, noticing any sensations or shifts in tension around the area.

EXERCISE 13: SPINAL TWISTS

Spinal twists are a gentle yet highly effective tension release exercise for increasing flexibility, releasing tension, and reducing stiffness along the entire spine. This exercise can contribute to overall spinal health, an increased range of motion, and more sustained feelings of well-being. You can use it for basic tension release or to help release spinal discomfort.

Instructions

You can do this exercise in a lying down or seated position with one simple alteration. Find a comfortable place with enough space to extend your legs out or twist your arms around. Prepare to use your breath to deepen this spinal twist.

Step 1: Lengthen Your Spine On The Inhale

Whether seated or lying down, take a deep breath in as you feel your spine lengthening. Imagine creating spaces between each vertebrae.

Step 2: Start With A Light Spinal Twist On The Exhale

If seated, place your right hand on your left knee and twist your spine as you exhale, looking over your left shoulder. If you're lying down flat on your back, bring your right

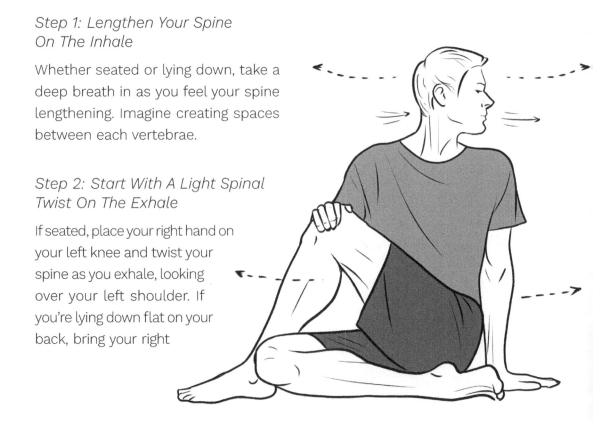

knee up and allow it to slowly drop across to the left as your shoulders stay flat on the floor.

Step 3: Feel The Rotation Of Your Spine

Allow your hand to pull you deeper into the stretch, but try not to strain. The stretch should feel releasing and comfortable.

Step 4: Hold For A Few Breaths

Hold the spinal twist as you continue to breathe. Breathe in deeply and use each exhale to release tension or deepen the twist.

Step 5: Repeat On The Other Side

Take a deep breath in and allow the exhale to soften the spinal twist. Bring your position back to the center slowly and repeat on the other side. Continue to alternate sides and tune into the tension you feel. If you feel a tight spot, take a deep breath in and use the exhale plus your hand to work through the tension.

EXERCISE 14: CAT-COW STRETCH

This fun somatic exercise, known as the cat-cow stretch, is popular in everyday yoga practices. It uses the alternating of two poses to balance spinal muscles and release tension along the upper back and neck in particular. This stretch increases blood flow to these areas, increasing flexibility and mobility along your entire spine.

Instructions

You can do this exercise on the floor or your bed. You will need to get on all fours with knees hip-width apart. Hold your neck in a neutral posture, facing down, and avoid hunching your shoulders.

Step 1: Inhale Deeply And Move Into Cow Pose

When you're ready, take a nice deep inhale through your nose as you arch your back and lift your head. You can also push your shoulder blades down, lift your gaze, and tilt your pelvis back.

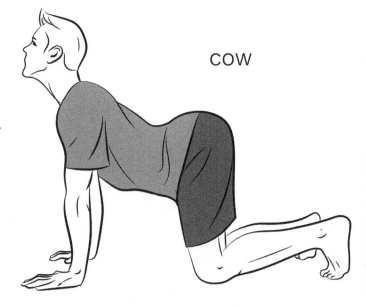

COW

Step 3: Hold

Hold the position for a full, long inhale and a short push at the end, feeling the muscles throughout your back almost squeezing.

Step 2: Move Into Cat Pose As You Exhale

As you release the exhale, move your body into the opposite position, rounding your back like a cat and dropping your chin, shoulders, and pelvis in.

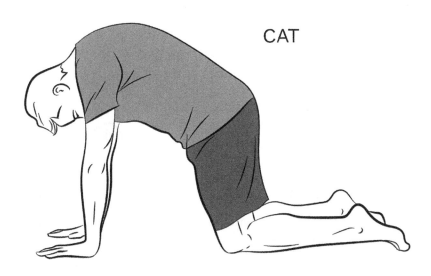

CAT

Step 3: Create A Flow Between The Poses

Continue to inhale and exhale now, creating a flow between the cat and cow poses. Allow the breath to deepen the stretch and circulate throughout your body.

Step 5: Explore Variations

As you become more comfortable with this exercise and have built up more spinal flexibility and mobility, you can explore some variations for a deeper tension release. Rather than just moving the pose up and down, you can circle your neck and hips to add more fluidity. This will further improve your flexibility and mobility, but only try it if it feels flowing and comfortable.

EXERCISE 15: ROLLING DOWN THE SPINE

The rolling down the spine somatic exercise is a gentle spinal release aimed at releasing tension along the spine while improving flexibility. It's an easy standing exercise that can be used as a simple warm-up stretch or full somatic exercise. It's a great opportunity to close your eyes and really sink into your body from a standing position.

Instructions

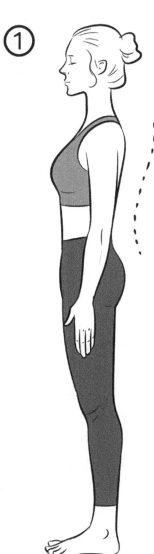

Find a private place where you can safely stand with enough room in front of you to bend forward and down. I recommend closing your eyes and using this exercise to soften your body.

Step 1: Straighten And Lengthen Your Posture

As you inhale deeply through your nose, straighten your posture and imagine a string pulling your spine up towards the ceiling from the top of your head.

Step 2: Exhale And Roll Your Body Down

On the exhale, start by dropping your chin, softening your shoulders inward, and rolling your body down until your upper body is completely folded over. You can bend your knees slightly to keep this exercise soft and relaxing.

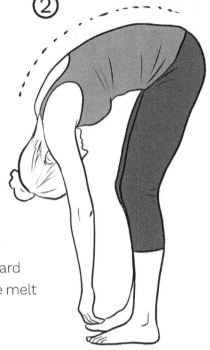

Step 3: Remain Standing And Relax Forward

As you hold your body up with your legs, allow your upper body to completely relax forward. Let your upper body hang softly toward the ground, feeling all the tension in your spine melt away. Take a couple of deep breaths in.

Step 4: Inhale And Roll Your Body Back Up Again

On the next big inhale, slowly roll your body back up again, starting at the hips, moving along the spine, and ending with your shoulders and chin. Repeat step 1 again.

Step 5: Repeat As Needed

Continue to roll your body down, resting in a forward fold for a moment, and rolling back up again as long as needed. Enjoy the sensations and softening you feel.

EXERCISE 16: CHILD'S POSE

The child's pose yoga position is a somatic exercise intended to fully release and relax the entire body. It is a resting position perfect for ending a somatic practice or completing before bed. This exercise promotes feelings of comfort within the body and mind, preparing the body for rest and release.

Instructions

Find a comfortable place on the floor or bed where you can kneel quietly. This is a kneeling, forward bend position that will release tension throughout your entire body, but mostly along your spine. Keep your breath flowing throughout and your eyes closed.

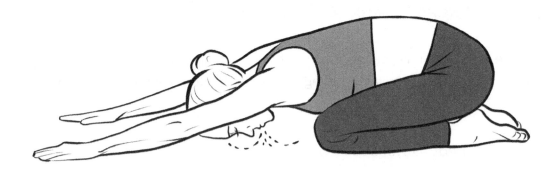

Step 1: Bring Feet Together And Knees Apart

As you kneel on the floor or bed, soften your feet beneath yourself and open the knees enough to make space for your body to fit between. Sit back on your heels comfortably.

Step 2: Fold Your Torso Over With Arms Stretched Forward

Bring your torso down between your knees with your arms stretched out in front of you. Allow your palms to pull your torso forward as you fully relax your upper body.

Step 3: Breathe Deeply And Relax

Spend as long as you need to in this pose, completely relaxing your entire body. You can sink your hips back or reposition yourself in any way that feels good.

Step 4: Explore Variations

Some variations of child's pose include resting your forehead on the ground in front of your knees to stretch out your neck muscles, bend your arms to rest your head on the backs of your hands instead, or bringing your arms back completely, allowing your shoulders and arms to soften fully. You can also increase the support under your body with a pillow or folded blanket to enable full relaxation.

Step 5: Exit Child's Pose Gently

This exercise requires a slow and gentle exit to maintain the softness and relaxation. To exit this pose, slowly walk your hands back, allowing your arms to lift your upper body out of the position. Take your time with this, and notice any sensations you feel.

EXERCISE 17: SEATED FORWARD BEND

The seated forward bend is a yoga position also known as Paschimottanasana. Although it is a simple stretch because it stretches both the back and legs, the spinal release is increased. Tight leg muscles, particularly the hamstrings, can contribute to lower back tightness. The seated forward bend relieves tension in all the muscles associated with spinal health, from head to toe.

Instructions

Find a comfortable place on the floor or a bed where you won't be disturbed. This stretch can be quite effective, so if the full stretch is too difficult, only bend as far forward as you're comfortable with.

Step 1: Sit Up Straight With Legs Straight Forward

Sit up with your back straight and your legs long in front of you.

Step 2: Inhale And Prepare To Stretch

Prepare to stretch by allowing the soles of your feet to flex up as if you were standing. Rest your hands on your knees and inhale deeply through your nose and into your belly.

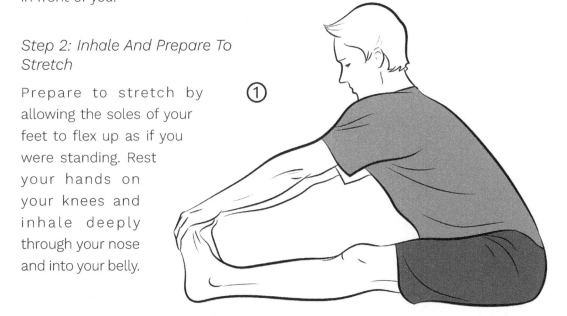

Step 3: Exhale And Bend Forward

Exhale slowly through your mouth as you bend forward. You can bend as far as is comfortable, challenging yourself enough to feel the stretch along your legs and spine.

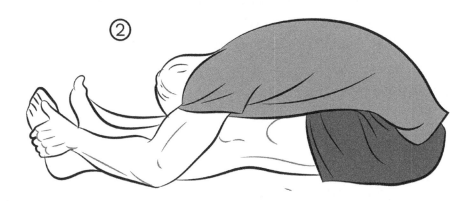

Step 4: Hold For A Few Breaths And Repeat

Hold the stretch for a few deep breaths. You can also use the breath to deepen the stretch if you'd like. Use your hands to gently pull you into a deeper bend. When you're reading, slowly return to normal, and repeat as necessary.

Step 5: Specify Your Variation

There are two variations to this forward bend: one that is more gentle and relaxing, and one that aims to deepen the stretch along your legs. You will likely already be in variation one, bending forward with a more rounded back. However, for a much deeper leg stretch try to keep your back straighter and bend only at the hips.

EXERCISE 18: STANDING FORWARD BEND

The standing forward bend is a powerful yoga pose also known as Uttanasana. It is a deeper and more difficult forward bend in comparison to the seated forward bend. Often, what intensifies these bends is the angle of the foot. Standing deepens the stretch significantly as your foot is fully flexed with gravity aiding the upper body's bend.

Instructions

Find a quiet place with enough space to bend forward fully with your body. You don't need to be able to touch your toes for this bend, simply stretch down as much as you're comfortable with.

Step 1: Stand Up Straight And Inhale Deeply

Prepare for your stretch by standing up straight and taking a long, slow inhale deep into your belly.

Step 2: Hinge Forward At The Hips

On the exhale, hinge forward at the hips while keeping your back straight. Lead with your chest and reach your hands down as you bend forward.

Step 3: Rest In the Stretch

Once you're as far forward as you can comfortably stretch, allow your hands to drop where they can

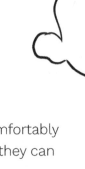

rest. If you can touch the floor with your fingertips, allow them to hang there. Or, if they are above the ground, rest them on the part of your legs or feet that they're closest to.

Step 4: Deepen With The Breath

As you breathe in and out, use your exhales to deepen the stretch. Continue to hinge forward at the hips and notice the changes in your hand position. You can also use your hands to help pull you forward by holding them behind your knees.

Step 5: Hold, Release, And Repeat

Hold your final position for a couple of breaths, tuning into the sensations throughout your body and release when you're ready. Feel the difference between the stretching tension and soft release. Repeat as necessary.

SECTION 4

MINDFULNESS
AND GROUNDING

EXERCISE 19: GROUNDING EXERCISES

There are various grounding exercises with the same goal in mind: to center your awareness and ground you into the present moment. These exercises are an excellent way to reconnect with the earth and reality as a whole, fostering a sense of inner stability, safety, and relaxation. These tools are most effective at reducing stress, relieving anxiety, and stabilizing mood.

Instructions

I'm going to share 3 simple grounding exercises with you. Find a quiet place to sit, stand, or lie down where you won't be disturbed. However, many of these exercises can be practiced in the heat of a stressful moment to help ground you.

Exercise 1: The Five Senses

For this exercise you will use your senses to ground you into the present moment: Sight, sound, smell, touch, and taste. Find 5 things in your environment you can see, 4 things you can hear, 3 things you can touch, 2 things you can smell, and 1 thing you can taste. As you engage with each sense, try to fully immerse yourself in the experience as you feel your awareness centering.

For example, if you're drinking a cup of coffee, notice the painting on your wall, the radio playing, the smell of the coffee, the feel of your sofa, and the taste of the sip you take.

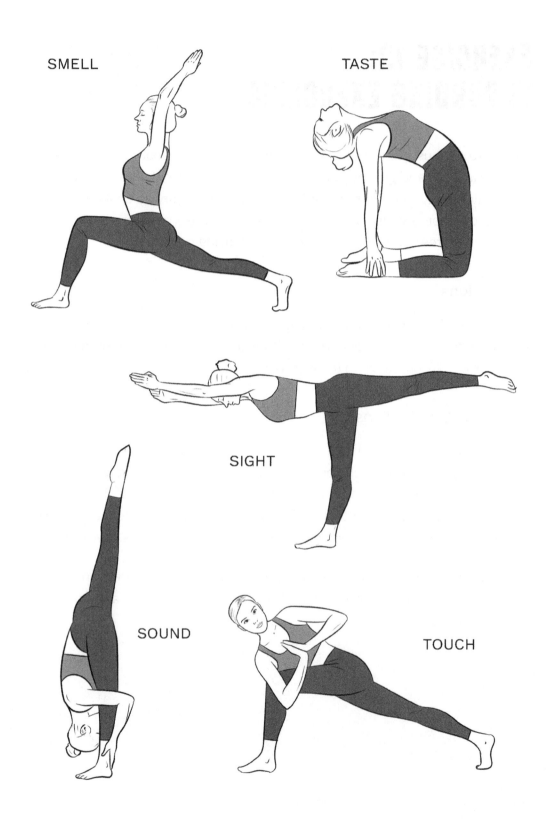

SMELL

TASTE

SIGHT

SOUND

TOUCH

Exercise 2: Barefoot Walking

The simplest way to ground a human being is by reconnecting with the earth. Because we often live very detached lives from nature, with technology, shoes, and supermarkets, feeling grounded in such an unnatural world is difficult. To reconnect with nature and physically ground your body to the earth, take off your shoes and walk barefoot.

As you walk, feel the sensations beneath your feet. Try to walk on various terrains to enhance this experience. Find some grass to walk on, then stones, then pavement. Feel the difference in sensations.

BAREFOOT WALKING

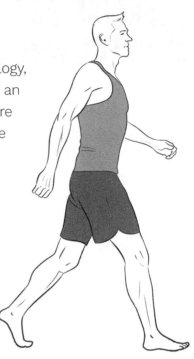

ROOTING VISUALIZATION

Exercise 3: Rooting Visualization

A rooting visualization is a great way to shift your perspective and feel grounded in the earth. As you're sitting or standing, close your eyes and visualize a root growing out the bottom of your feet and down into the earth. As the root grows down, visualize the core of the earth glowing a color of your choice. When your root reaches the core of the earth, the color spreads up your roots and through your body. Tune into any sensations you might feel.

EXERCISE 20: MINDFUL WALKING

Mindful walking is a mindfulness exercise that encourages contemplation, heightened awareness, and relaxation. It takes something most of us do every day and transforms it into a time of peaceful gratitude. Mindful walking cultivates mindfulness through intentional, focused walking which will allow you to more easily ground into the present when needed.

Instructions

Find a place where you can safely walk without obstacles. You can alternate between open and closed eyes if possible, deepening the experience.

Step 1: Start At A Standstill

Stand still and upright for a moment, taking deep breaths to help you center. Take a moment to observe your surroundings, engaging each of your senses if possible and heightening your awareness. Continue to breathe deeply throughout the exercise.

Step 2: Set An Intention

Decide on an intention for your mindful walk. It can be something like finding clarity on a topic, practicing focus, stress reduction, or simply enjoyment.

Step 3: Begin Walking Slowly

Bring your awareness to your body now and start walking slowly. Allow each step to be focused and intentional.

Step 4: Focus On Every Sensation

Allow your awareness to be fully present in each sensation. Feel the soles of your feet flexing and arching. Feel the weight of your foot as it swings forward. Feel your arms gently swaying. Tune into the experience and be as present and grounded as possible. Notice every sensation of walking that you normally don't truly experience.

Step 5: Mindfully Conclude

When you're ready to conclude the exercise, slowly bring your awareness back from your body and into your environment again. Focus on the sights, sounds, smells, and anything else you can. Allow your breath to return to normal, and take some time to reflect on the experience.

EXERCISE 21: EYE PALMING

The eyes are a common place for tension to build. But because they are also responsible for sight, eye palming works to relax us in two very effective ways. By covering the eyes with our palms, we not only help relieve tension and pressure but we cut off visual stimuli, which can help calm the mind.

Instructions

You can do this exercise sitting, standing, or lying down, provided you are in a safe place. This exercise is best used during the day to help maintain a sense of calm, but you can use it whenever needed.

Step 1: Prepare Your Hands

Rub your palms together to create some friction, the warmth will produce a more comforting experience. Cup your hands gently to create a slight hollow in closed hands.

Step 2: Cover your Eyes

Bring your palms up to your eyes, covering them as much as possible without applying too much pressure. The hollows of your palms should create a small space above each eye so you can open them. If you're struggling to cut out all the light, adjust your hands as needed.

Step 3: Take Deep Breathes

Start taking deep breaths to bring a sense of calm and relaxation.

Step 4: Hold And Feel The Sensation Of Darkness

Hold your hands in place for a few deep breaths and allow yourself to feel the sensation of darkness on your eyes. Soften the tension in your brow and allow your eyes to rest.

Step 5: Remove Slowly And Gently

When you're ready, slowly soften your hands and allow the light back in. Gently open your eyes and take note of how your eyes feel. They will likely feel refreshed and clear.

EXERCISE 22: SOMATIC VISUALIZATION

Somatic visualization is a powerful tool promoting relaxation and tension release with nothing but the power of the mind. It involves putting imagery around our tension to help us let go and release. Practiced regularly, this somatic practice can increase body awareness, reduce stress, and improve your sense of well-being.

Instructions

Find a comfortable place to sit or lie down where you won't be disturbed. However, lying down is recommended. Close your eyes and breathe deeply throughout this exercise.

Step 1: Start With A Body Scan

As you breathe deeply and hold your eyes closed, proceed with a body scan. Pause to acknowledge any areas of tension or discomfort.

Step 2: Give Your Tension A Color And Shape

Start with one area of tension or discomfort if there are many. Give your tension or discomfort a shape, color, size, or any other visualization that makes sense to you. For example, you could see your tension as a dark mist, a tight knot of rope, a heavy cloud, or a murky puddle.

Step 3: Visually Release The Tension

Holding your awareness on this area of tension, choose a way to visually release the tension in a way that makes sense with its shape. For example, you can visualize the tight knot becoming untangled, the dark mist escaping with every exhale, and the murky puddle being washed clean by a stream of water. Whatever feels right for you, visualize the tension releasing.

Step 4: Tune Into Sensations

As you visualize the tension leaving your body, try to feel the physical release. Tune into any sensations you feel, and imagine the physical tension softening and fading as you release.

Step 5: Repeat For Each Area

If there are multiple areas of tension or discomfort, you can repeat the steps for each area. However, if you are pressed for time or there are too many areas, simply visualize each area and release simultaneously. For example, if all your tension is dark mist, visualize your breath collecting the mist on the inhale and releasing it on the exhale.

EXERCISE 23: YOGA SUN SALUTATIONS

Sun salutations are a series of yoga poses completed in what is known as a flow with the intention of energizing the body and improving the mind-body connection. There are 12 positions in total which together warm up, stretch, and strengthen the entire body.

Instructions

Find a comfortable place where you will have enough room to stretch out. You can either alternate breathing per pose, or you can pause in each position allowing the breath to flow.

Position 1: Mountain Pose

Stand tall with feet hip-width apart and bring your palms together in front of your chest.

Position 2: Upward Salute

Keeping your palms together, inhale deeply, and reach your palms up above your head.

Position 3: Forward Fold

As you exhale, fold forward at the hips, dropping your hands down onto your shins or feet.

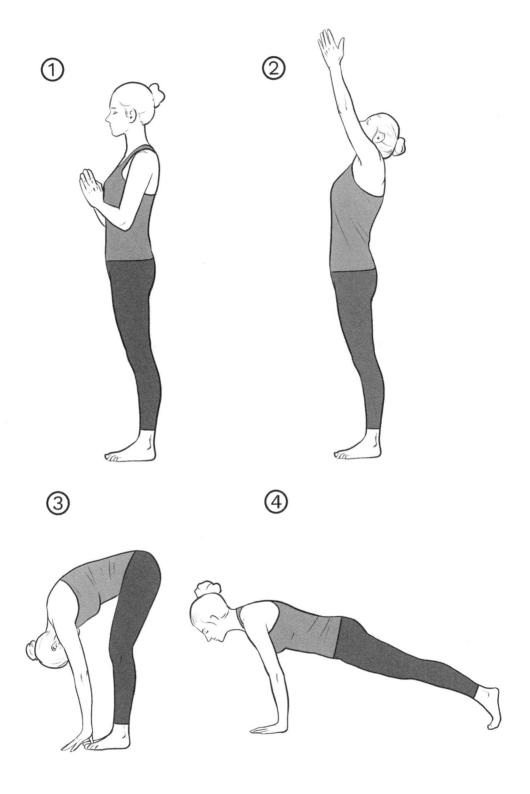

Position 4: Plank Position

Bend your knees, press your weight onto your palms, and step back into a plank position.

Position 5: Upward Facing Dog

Move from your toes onto the backs of your feet, then dip your hips and arch your back.

Position 6: Downward Facing Dog

Step onto your toes pressing your weight back with your palms. Drop your head and lift your hips.

Position 7: Forward Fold

Step both feet forward back to standing, with your upper body bent over in a forward fold again.

Position 8: Upward Salute

Inhale deeply, lifting your arms high above your head and placing your palms back together.

Position 9: Mountain Pose

Slowly lower your palms back in front of your chest and finish in mountain pose. Repeat 1-9.

SECTION 5

GRACEFUL MOVEMENTS
FOR FLEXIBILITY

EXERCISE 24: TAI CHI MOVEMENTS

Tai Chi is an ancient form of Martial Arts, originating in China. The movements are slow, smooth, and deliberate to encourage balance and calm throughout the body and mind. This practice promotes mind-body awareness, relaxation, and overall well-being. There are many movements within the practice ranging from balancing positions, arm movements, and steady postures.

Instructions

Find a peaceful area to practice, where you can move freely without obstruction. I'm going to share an introduction to one of the most popular Tai Chi movement sequences known as Grasp the Sparrows tail.

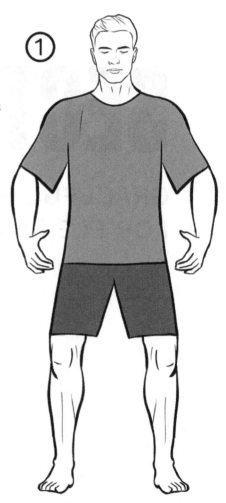

Position 1: Starting Position

Standing in a relaxed and upright position, step your feet out shoulder-width apart. Tuck your pelvis in, bend your knees slightly, and keep your spine straight. Bring your awareness to your breath, inhaling and exhaling slowly.

Position 2: Ward Off

Start with the left leg, you will come back to this step after position 5 and redo the sequence with the opposite leg and arm. Step your left leg to the side, turn your torso with it, and shift your balance onto your left leg. Expand your arms in a circular motion, leading with the left arm.

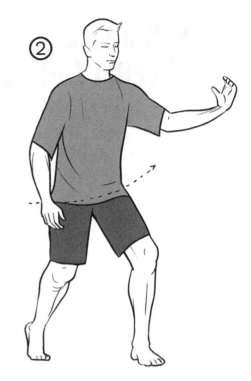

Position 3: Roll Back

Continue the circular motion of your arms, bringing both back towards your body and to the other side while simultaneously shifting your weight back to your other leg.

Position 4: Press

Now bring your hands together into the center of your chest, shifting your weight back onto your front leg and pressing the hands forward.

Position 5: Push

From the press position, round the hands back toward the stomach with palms facing outward as you shift your weight into a more centered position. Then shift your weight forward again as you push your palms forward and slightly up together.

Position 6: Pivot To The Other Side And Repeat

Shift your weight and pivot to the center, with your arms in the middle. Repeat on the other side.

EXERCISE 25: BUTTERFLY POSE

The butterfly yoga pose, also known as Baddha Konasana in Sanskrit, is a seated hip opening pose that increases flexibility and mobility in the hips and groin areas. Along with releasing tension in the pelvic region, it is also known to have a calming effect on the nervous system, promoting relaxation and well-being.

Instructions

This is a seated position, best practiced in a quiet and comfortable environment. If the position is too difficult, you can use yoga blocks or cushions underneath your knees to support your legs.

Step 1: Sit Up Straight With Legs Extended

Take a moment to sit up straight with your legs extended in front of you. Take a couple of deep breaths to center yourself. Keep your back straight throughout this exercise.

Step 2: Bend Your Knees And Bring Feet Together

When you're ready, bend your knees and bring the soles of your feet together. Your knees should be resting in this position in order to stretch and open the hips.

Step 3: Hold Your Feet

Hold your feet with your hands, using them to help bring your feet closer in toward yourself. This should deepen the stretch and prepare you for step 4.

Step 4: Deepen With Butterfly Wings

If you're comfortable deepening this stretch, gently rock your knees up and down, as if flapping butterfly wings.

Step 5: Release Slowly

Enjoy this tension-relieving exercise for as long as you'd like. However, when you're ready to finish, release your feet from the position slowly.

EXERCISE 26: CROSS-CRAWL EXERCISE

This fun somatic exercise, known as the cross-crawl exercise, is a coordinated movement that uses the entire body to engage the left and right hemispheres of the brain. The cross-crawl is an easy and effective way to enhance coordination and cognitive function by helping to balance and tone the nervous system.

Instructions

Find a quiet place where you can stand up straight and complete this exercise. It can be completed on the ground if you have sliding pads to place beneath your knees and hands, but standing works all the same.

Step 1: Stand Up Straight

Stand up straight with shoulders back and face forward. Take a deep breath and engage your core as you begin.

Step 2: Touch Your Right Knee To Left Elbow

Lift your right knee up towards your chest while simultaneously bringing your left arm up with your palm facing forward. Then bring your left elbow down to touch your right knee. This should twist your torso slightly. Keep your your core engaged and balance steady.

Step 3: Return To Neutral Position

Return your right leg to the ground and left arm gently to your side as you stand up straight again for a moment.

Step 4: Alternate To The Other Knee And Elbow

Alternate to the other knee and elbow, bringing your left knee and right arm up, before touching elbow to knee.

Step 5: Repeat In A Rhythmic Fashion

Repeat the alternating movements in a fluid, rhythmic fashion. It should look almost as if you were crawling in the air. Bring your awareness to the sensations through your body and take note of how you feel. Repeat for a few minutes or so before coming to a gentle standstill.

EXERCISE 27: ARM STRETCHING AND RELEASING

There are many effective arm stretching and releasing exercises designed to release tension, stretch muscles, increase flexibility, and improve well-being. Tension in the neck and arms can create stiffness, nerve pain, and even pinched nerves. Practicing arm stretching and releasing regularly can help you avoid chronic problems and damage that may inhibit functioning.

Instructions

Find a comfortable place to sit down with a straight back and neutral head position. I'm going to share 3 highly effective arm stretches and releases that you can add to your somatic practice for a more targeted release.

Release 1: Neck And Shoulder Rolls

Starting with your shoulders, sit up straight and roll your shoulders forward repeatedly. Breathe in deeply throughout. Switch to rolling the shoulders backward for a couple of rounds.

Next, drop your chin down to your chest and roll your head from left to right. You can also roll slightly past your shoulder on either side to stretch the sides of the front of your neck. Feel the stretch releasing throughout your shoulders, decolletage, and neck.

Release 2: Tricep Stretch

The triceps are a muscle we are not often aware of, making them a common place for tension to be stored. Stretching one arm at a time, reach the arm up above your head and bend the elbow allowing your hand to drop gently behind your back. Your elbow should be pointing toward the ceiling.

Next, take your opposite hand and place it on your elbow. Use the opposite hand to pull the elbow inward and backward slightly, feeling a nice stretch along the tricep. Repeat on the other arm.

Release 3: Eagle Arms Stretch

Reach both arms forward, crossing them at the elbow. Now turn both palms to face each other, bringing them together in a twisted arm position. Hold your hands together and lift them above your head. Hold the stretch and feel your arms and shoulders getting a nice release.

You can use this stretch behind your back, lifting your arms up to stretch and squeeze your shoulder blades. For either stretch, alternate which hand is on the top.

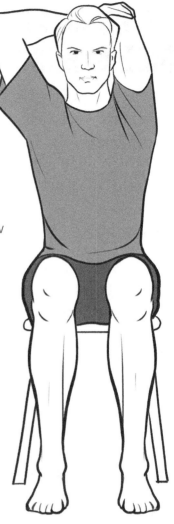

EXERCISE 28: SIDE BENDS

Side bends are a great addition to any stretching or somatic routine to target tension release and increased flexibility in the sides of the torso. This exercise works to stretch and strengthen the obliques and intercostal muscles for improved lateral flexibility.

Instructions

Find somewhere you can comfortably stand and extend your arms out to your sides. You can also do seated side bends if necessary.

Step 1: Stand Up Straight And Inhale

Stand with your spine straight and posture neutral. Inhale deeply through your nose, reaching your arms out to either side of your body like a starfish.

Step 2: Bend At The Hip And Reach Down To The Left

Starting on your left side, bend your torso over to the left at the hips. Keep your gaze forward and drop your left arm down, sliding it along your left leg as you stretch. You can keep your right arm extended into the air or deepen the stretch by bringing it over your head to the left.

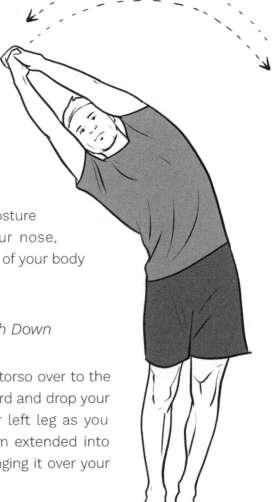

Step 3: Feel The Stretch And Hold

Continue to breathe deeply as you hold the stretch. Tune into the sensations of the stretch, feeling any tension or discomfort before releasing.

Step 4: Release And Straighten Up Slowly

Soften the stretch and slowly bring your torso back up with arms extended at either side again. Feel the contrast between the stretch and relaxation. Notice the softness and any other sensations you feel.

Step 5: Repeat On The Other Side

Repeat the steps on the other side, stretching your right arm down your right side to stretch the left side of your torso. Repeat on both sides for a minute or so, holding, stretching, and breathing deeply for a relaxing release.

EXERCISE 29: KNEE-TO-CHEST STRETCH

The knee-to-chest stretch is a simple stretch with a lot of benefits. Lying down on the ground and stretching one knee to the chest at a time offers a tremendous tension release in the hips and lower back. This exercise can improve flexibility and promote relaxation. It is the perfect choice for those who spend a lot of time sitting.

Instructions

Find a comfortable place to lie flat on your back with your legs extended. You can complete this exercise on your bed, but a floor may provide some extra tension release as the muscles massage against a harder surface.

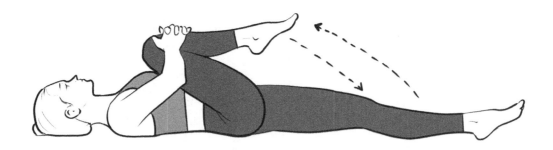

Step 1: Sink Into The Starting Position

Lying flat on your back with legs extended straight down and arms relaxed by your sides, take a couple of deep breaths, feeling your body press into the ground.

Step 2: Bend One Knee And Hold

Slowly bend one knee, bringing it up towards your chest. Use your hand to hold it in place and deepen the stretch. You can hold the leg at the shin or thigh, wherever is most comfortable.

Step 3: Slowly Lower And Switch

Lower the raised leg slowly back onto the ground, taking note of the release you feel. Raise your other leg up towards your chest and repeat.

Step 4: Knee To Chest Variation

You can take this stretch further by bringing both legs up to your chest at the same time. Hold with your hands and if you're comfortable with it, you can rock slightly from side to side for a nice deep hip and lower back release.

Step 5: Feel The Sensations

Take a moment to close your eyes and sink into the hip stretch. This exercise is best practiced slowly, allowing the weight of your body to melt away tension. Continue to breathe deeply and tune into any sensations you feel. When you're ready, sink back into the starting position to rest for a moment.

EXERCISE 30: FIGURE-EIGHT HIP MOVEMENTS

Often used in dance routines, but also an all-around lower body release, figure-eight hip movements are fluid and fun. The smooth swaying motion engages muscles around the hip joints helping to strengthen them and promote a full range of motion. This exercise reduces tension in the pelvis, spine, and hips while boosting a sense of well-being.

Instructions

This movement is completed in a standing position with feet about hip width apart. Find somewhere you can comfortably swing your hips and have fun with this exercise.

Step 1: Prepare To Move

Standing up straight with your feet about hip-width apart, place your hands on your hips and face forward.

Step 2: Begin The Figure Of Eight

To begin the figure of eight, turn your hips to face the right without moving your feet. From this position lead the figure of eight with your left hip, alternating between the two hips as we go.

Step 3: Draw The Figure Of Eight

Draw a figure of eight, imagining that the cross point of the eight is at your center of gravity. Pull your hips from left to right in a figure of eight, turning your hips to face either side slightly as you go.

Step 4: Get Into The Swing Of It

If you're comfortable completing this movement, allow yourself to get into a flow. Let your hips swing lightly through the figure of eight, feeling the fluidity and release.

Step 5: Have Fun With It

Allow yourself to have fun with this exercise. Notice any shifts in your mobility and mood as you go. Tune into any sensations or cues of relaxation. This is an exercise that can easily boost your mood and feelings of well-being.

EXERCISE 31: PSOAS RELEASE EXERCISE

The psoas is a deep-seated muscle connecting the lumbar spine to the femur.[4] It is a common place for tension to build and is a difficult place to find release. Most regular stretches for the back and hips do not fully expand or relax this muscle. These psoas release exercises can target the muscle directly, reducing lower back discomfort and improving hip flexibility.

Instructions

Find a comfortable place where you have enough space to complete these exercises. I'm going to share three of the most effective on-the-ground psoas release exercises.

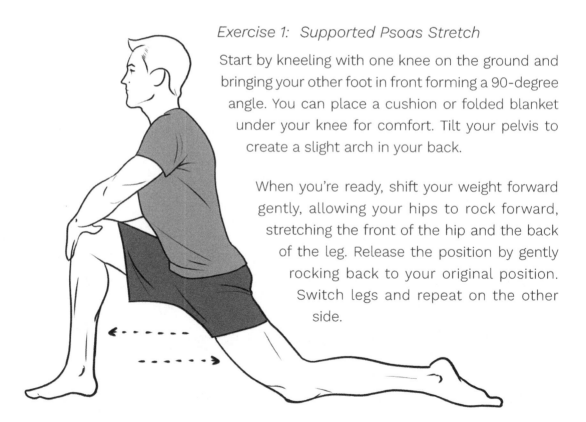

Exercise 1: Supported Psoas Stretch

Start by kneeling with one knee on the ground and bringing your other foot in front forming a 90-degree angle. You can place a cushion or folded blanket under your knee for comfort. Tilt your pelvis to create a slight arch in your back.

When you're ready, shift your weight forward gently, allowing your hips to rock forward, stretching the front of the hip and the back of the leg. Release the position by gently rocking back to your original position. Switch legs and repeat on the other side.

Exercise 2: Hip Raises For Psoas Release

Start by lying on your back with your knees bent and feet on the ground. Keep your feet in line with your hips and raise your pelvis off the ground. Slowly raise and lower your pelvis off the ground to engage the glute muscles and stretch the front of your hips.

To deepen the psoas release of this exercise, complete about a minute or two of hip raises before slowly moving to a standing position. Once standing, place your hands on your lower back, and stretch your hips forward. You should feel a nice release in your lower back area.

Exercise 3: Active Psoas Release

Start in a lunge position, placing your knee on the ground with your other foot in front at a 90-degree angle. When you're ready, slide your knee back into a high lunge position. You can distribute your weight across the knee, foot, and lower leg. Place this back leg on a folded blanket for more support if needed.

To activate the release, engage your core and tuck your pelvis under slightly. Gently rock your hips forward and back against your front leg feeling the release along the front of your back leg and hip. Slowly come back to neutral and switch legs. Repeat on the other side.

EXERCISE 32: LATERAL NECK STRETCH

This neck stretch, known as the lateral neck stretch, does exactly what you would expect – stretching and releasing the lateral muscles of the neck. The muscles along the side of the neck include some shoulder muscles such as the trapezius. This stretch can relieve tension, increase flexibility, and reduce stiffness in all of these muscles simultaneously.

Instructions

Find a comfortable place to sit for this stretch. You can do it on the edge of a bed, on the floor, or at your work desk. It's a great stretch to do throughout the day helping to release tension and prevent tension build up.

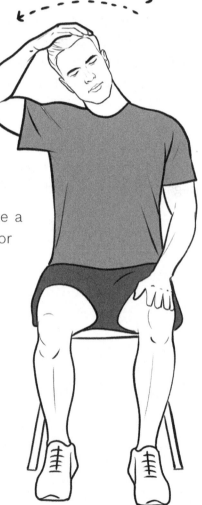

Step 1: Sit Up Straight And Inhale

Take a moment to sit up straight. You can take a couple of deep breaths in this position first, or simply inhale deeply and move ont the stretch.

Step 2: Tilt Your Head To One Side

On the exhale, drop your head slowly to one side, almost reaching it toward your shoulder. Avoid lifting your shoulders, keep them square throughout. Allow the weight of your head to stretch the muscles.

Step 3: Slowly Release And Repeat

When you're ready, slowly lift your head back to a neutral position. Take a deep breath in and repeat on the other side.

Step 4: Deepen The Stretch

To deepen this stretch, use your hand to apply slight pressure onto the side of your head. If you are tilting your head to the left, bring your left hand over and onto the right side near your ear. Simply rest your hand here to deepen the stretch. Avoid applying too much pressure.

Step 5: Notice The Sensations

As you stretch your lateral neck muscles, notice any tension or stiffness you feel. Use your breath to release tension, and notice if your head continues to drop down as the muscles release. You can take note of your progress by monitoring your stiffness or range of motion.

EXERCISE 33: SELF-MASSAGE

Self-massage is a somatic practice that allows you to directly target and focus on relieving tension in specific muscles. Using your hands or massage tools, you can apply pressure to your muscles and work out the tension or stiffness. Self-massage is a great way to relax, foster a stronger mind-body connection, and feel empowered to take care of your tension.

Instructions

You can sit or lie down for this exercise, adjusting your position as you massage different muscles throughout your body.

Step 1: Deep Breathing

It's easier to release muscle tension through massage when you are in a relaxed frame of mind. Take a few deep diaphragmatic breaths before you begin.

Step 2: Complete A Body Scan

To help you decide where your body needs massaging most, you can use a body scan meditation. Scan your awareness through your body, taking note of any areas that feel tense or uncomfortable.

Step 3: Massage With Your Hands

Start massaging the tense area you are working on with your hands. You can use your fingertips, palms, or knuckles to stroke the area. Some common massage strokes include circular motions, long strokes, and kneading. You can apply as much pressure as you're comfortable with.

Step 4: Tips To Deepen Self-Massage

To achieve a better result with self-massage, you can try:

- Using massage oils or lotion.

- Implementing massage tools like foam rollers or massage balls.

- Move intuitively, adjusting positions and pressure to what feels best.

Step 5: Lean Into Relaxation

The more relaxed you can become during self-massage, the easier it will be to release tension. Lean into relaxation by closing your eyes, tuning into the sensations, and centering yourself into the present moment.

SECTION 6

BALANCE AND FOCUS

EXERCISE 34: BALANCING ON ONE FOOT

The balancing act of trying to keep steady on one foot is a good indication of your proprioception and coordination. However, it can also be improved with practice. As your balance improves so will your overall proprioception, focus, and stability within your body. Balancing on one foot is a fun somatic practice to work on improved balance.

Instructions

To practice balancing on one foot, you will need to find a comfortable, sturdy place to stand. However, if you need assistance, you can use the back of a chair or stand near a wall for support.

Step 1: Stand Up Tall

Start by standing up tall with feet about hip-width apart. Take a few deep breaths in and decide on an arm position. Hands on the hips is a great start.

Step 2: Shift Weight Onto One Leg

When you're ready, shift your entire weight onto one foot, lifting the other off the ground slightly.

Step 3: Engage Core And Balance

Engage your core and place your foot where you're comfortable. This can be resting on the other foot for an easier variation or held up at your shin with the knee bent. Hold this position and balance for up to 30 seconds.

Step 4: Switch Legs

When you're ready, switch positions to the other side. Keep your arm and feet position the same for the other side for an even sense of balance. Repeat on steps 2 & 3.

Step 5: Challenge Yourself

You can repeat the exercise as is for a few minutes. However, if you'd like to challenge yourself and further improve your balance you can:

- Close your eyes.

- Stand without an aid.

- Hold arms out to the side.

- Stand on a yoga block.

As you try new ways to balance, monitor your progress and see what a difference it makes.

EXERCISE 35:
SOMATIC EMPATHY EXERCISE

The somatic empathy exercise is arguably one of the most important somatic practices for emotional trauma release or regulation. It is an exercise where you can explore the complex interplay between emotions and the body, learning to connect emotions and sensations. It's important to withhold a strong sense of self-compassion and curiosity when practicing to improve your sense of well-being and self-care.

Instructions

You can choose to sit or lie down for this exercise, finding a comfortable place where you won't be disturbed. Take a few deep breaths to prepare and get started.

Step 1: Reflect On Your Emotions

Close your eyes as you breathe deeply. Take a moment to notice and reflect on any emotions you feel. Whatever emotions you feel, such as anxiety, anger, joy, or peace, try to put a label on them if possible.

Step 2: Complete A Body Scan

Next, keeping your eyes closed, complete a body scan exercise. Scan your awareness from head to toe, taking note of any sensations you feel. Simply acknowledge the sensations and move on.

Step 3: Connect Emotions With Sensations

Without judgment, take a moment to decipher which sensations belong to your emotions. Some sensations may have nothing to do with how you feel. However, others may be present because of the emotion.

Step 4: Release And Let Go

Once you've practiced somatic empathy, it's important to release and let go of any negative emotions and tension. Do what feels right, such as any somatic movements, deep breathing, or mindful visualizations.

Step 5: Reflect On The Change

Take a moment to reflect on how you feel both emotionally and physically. Notice the changes and compare the sensations to how you felt before. You can also use this time to journal down which sensations you discovered were connected to which emotions.

6

YOUR PERSONALIZED SOMATIC EXERCISE PLAN

10 Minutes Per Day For A Harmonized Nervous System

"Success is the sum of small efforts repeated day in and day out."

– Robert Collier

Think of a set of guitar strings stretching along the body from the head to the bridge. Every time the strings are played, they loosen a little. The strings are eventually stressed out of tune and need a tune-up to sound great again. The human nervous system is much the same.

When we experience stressors in our lives, our nervous system takes a hit. But if we haven't tuned it up in a while, the stressors we could once tolerate create an unorchestrated reaction within us. When we don't have nervous system harmony, stress can create chaos in the body.

But just like a guitar, with regular maintenance and tuning, the nervous system can strengthen to the point of withstanding stress. When the strings are well-oiled and tightly tuned, the sound can easily bounce off of them. A regular somatic practice is enough to tune up the nervous system so stress can simply bounce off of it.

10 minutes a day is all you need for a harmonized nervous system in the long term. Quality and regularity are far more beneficial than time spent. In this chapter, I'm going to guide you through creating a somatic exercise plan that is tailored to your nervous system. Each of us has different stressors, different bodies, and unique somatic responses. A tailored plan will make sure that the 10 minutes you spend doing somatics daily are worth it.

WHERE TO START

To choose the right exercises for your exercise plan, you'll need to get to the bottom of what your needs are. This is an opportunity to reflect back on the body scan you did in Chapter 2. However, you can complete a more recent or thorough body scan right now to help you gain more insights into your physical and psychological well-being. There will be a new outline for you to fill in in your Workbook.

When you're ready, there is a questionnaire in your Workbook with questions that will help you further evaluate your physical and emotional state. Please take a moment to fill those out before continuing.

Now that you're clear on your unique and targeted needs, the next step toward a complete 10-minute somatic exercise plan is to set goals. There is space in your Workbook to write down your goals. Some tips to help you define clear and achievable objectives include:

- Be specific and clear.

- Choose measurable benchmarks.

- Have realistic expectations.

- Assign a realistic time frame to each goal.

- Ensure they align with your overall well-being.

- Be open to adjusting them if necessary.

- Celebrate your successes, no matter how small.

Take a moment to fill out your goals in your Workbook. Choose 2 easily attainable goals, 2 more challenging goals, and 1 main goal or objective.

CHOOSING EXERCISES

This is the most personal part of your exercise plan. Which exercises you choose to do daily will come down to a few important factors, including your:

- Needs: Reflect on your self-assessment and goals.

- Focus: What is your main goal? For example improved well-being, mobility, or relaxation.

- Mobility: Which exercises work best for your mobility levels.

- Environment: How much space or privacy do you have to work with

- Comfort: Which exercises are you psychologically comfortable practicing.

In your Workbook, there is a checklist of the 35 exercises you learned in Chapter 5. Consider choosing up to 10 exercises on the list. Depending on your overall goal and target areas, you can choose exercises from each section or fine-tune your selection to just one or two sections. If you're unsure, take some time to go back to Chapter 5 and feel which exercises are right for you.

CREATING YOUR PLAN

Once you've chosen up to 10 exercises, consider the time you'd like to spend on each. You may end up choosing just 5 of the 10 exercises for a consistent daily plan, or you can alternate between the exercises on different days. Hypothetically, you could even practice all 35 exercises by sectioning off the exercises into a 7-day plan of just 10 minutes a day. It's completely up to you.

The important thing to aim for with a daily somatic practice is balance. If you're going to complete the same set of exercises daily, make sure to complete them in an order that compliments one another. For example

- 1-minute warm-up body scan

- 5 minutes of seated somatic exercises (3 exercises)

- 2 minutes of standing somatic exercises (1 exercise)

- 1-minute cool-down visualization and breathing

This simple layout is a great way to create a nice flowing routine with a beginning and an end. You might choose to start and end your daily workout in the same way while alternating the exercises in between. To end up with a layout like this, you could choose exercises in the following way:

- 1-minute warm-up: One exercise to center the mind (ie. Somatic breath counting).

- 6 minutes of main exercises: this could be 3 exercises of your choice (2 minutes each).

- 2-minute release: A releasing exercise (ie. shaking or releasing visualization).

- 1-minute cool-down: One final exercise to process and integrate the experience (ie. Diaphragmatic breathing).

If you are someone who prefers a more flexible schedule, you could decide on a layout like the one above and choose a selection of exercises you could alternate between during the main portion of your daily somatic workout. Use the space in your Workbook to create a daily somatic exercise plan.

For example, if you have 10 main exercises that work great for you, you could warm up with a body scan and intuitively choose the 3 exercises that you feel are most needed for the day. Provided that you only spend 2 minutes on each exercise, you can keep your workout within the 10-minute slot you've allocated for your somatic practice.

MONITOR YOUR PROGRESS

The shifts and progress felt after practicing somatic exercises can range from subtle to life-changing. However, most of the time, it's the small changes that add up to life-changing results. Keeping track of these small changes will help you to look back and recognize how far you've come. Monitoring your progress and celebrating the smallest improvements will be incredibly encouraging. Some things you can do to actively recognize your progress include:

- Journaling: Take notes of your sessions. Mark down any new sensations, thoughts, experiences or changes you notice. This can mean a quick written check-in before and after each session.

- Identify markers of progress: These can include flexibility, pain, mood, or psychological changes.

- Identify increased awareness: Look out for signs of an improved mind-body awareness such as improved appetite, quicker recognition of emotions, or an improved ability to identify target areas.

- Talking to a friend or doctor: feedback from friends, relatives, or your doctor is a great resource for tracking progress. You could also reach out to them for help when facing a challenge to recieve the necessary support.

- Checking off and setting goals: setting small attainable goals is another great way to track progress as you can check them off your list as you go, taking note of your past goals and setting new ones for continued encouragement and motivation.

There are pages provided for a week of somatic journaling to help you track your progress. Keeping track of your progress is also a great way to know when you need to change things. If you follow your somatic exercise plan and don't see results for some time, it might be a sign that you're not feeling challenged enough. This is an opportunity to reevaluate your daily 10-minute workout strategy. Maybe there's an exercise that you could switch out or deepen. Give yourself the benefit of the doubt and try out exercises you previously felt were out of your comfort zone.

The truth about progress is that sometimes what once worked starts to feel ineffective because you've made more progress than you've realized! If this happens, simply try out some more difficult variations of the exercises you love or switch up your plan completely.

Our bodies shift and change constantly. Be sure to check in with yourself regularly to make sure your goals are still aligned with your changing needs. If a specific problem you had starts to resolve and new areas of tension emerge, start at the beginning of this chapter and have fun creating a new 10-minute somatic exercise plan tailored to your new goals and needs.

The nervous system, like strings on a guitar, can be tuned up to better handle stress – this is known as a toned nervous system. The most important thing to remember about a somatic practice is consistency. If your nervous system feels out of tune, it's important to commit to spending time within yourself daily, even when you feel good.

Sometimes, a guitar can still function and sound good when the strings are a day away from needing a retune. So rather than waiting for dysregulation, keep your nervous system strong and toned with daily practice.

CONCLUSION

Healing is one of the most challenging yet rewarding journeys one can face. Both mental or physical healing journeys require the other to see long-term progress. Because of the mind-body connection, physical healing takes mental harmony, and vice versa. We are complex beings made up of an intricate entanglement of physical and mental processes. You can't have one without the other. Knowing that is a superpower.

When you build a strong mind-body connection, paired with your deep desire to be well, you become an empowered self-healer. You access one of the most miraculous mechanisms in existence – the mind-body connection. And because it is something that has been overlooked in most other healing modalities, it's what makes somatics so special.

I love the thought that during this book, you most likely stopped what you were doing, got up from where you were lying down or sitting, and tried out at least one of the 35 somatic exercises. I love that you felt compelled to move your body, tune into it, and *feel*. That is true action. And as I like to remind myself and others, healing takes action.

You have to make a choice and do something about your pain, trauma, or stress. It's not likely to go away on its own, and all I can wish for is that since reading this book, you feel more empowered to take the necessary action to relieve your struggles. You deserve so much to be comfortable and safe in your body. Let somatic practice guide the way.

REFERENCES

1. https://www.nichd.nih.gov/health/topics/neuro/conditioninfo/functions#:~:text=The%20nervous%20system%20plays%20a,Brain%20growth%20and%20development

2. https://greatergood.berkeley.edu/article/item/how_to_grow_the_good_in_your_brain

3. https://www.ncbi.nlm.nih.gov/pmc/articles/PMC4427060/#:~:text=Sighs%20monitor%20changes%20in%20brain,thereby%20become%20critical%20for%20survival

4. https://www.ncbi.nlm.nih.gov/books/NBK535418/#:~:text=The%20psoas%20muscle%20is%20among,to%20form%20the%20iliopsoas%20muscle

WORKBOOK 1

SOMATIC EXERCISES
FOR NERVOUS SYSTEM REGULATION

35 Beginner – Intermediate Techniques
To Reduce Anxiety & Tone Your Vagus Nerve In
Under 10 Minutes A Day

NOTES

WELCOME

I'm so glad you've made the decision to use the Workbook. It shows you're taking this seriously, and it leads me to believe that you'll not only do the exercises, but you'll experience the benefits this work has to offer. That makes me so pleased.

This Workbook will complement what you've read in 'Somatic Exercises.' You'll discover even more about how your mind and body can work together in harmonious ways. This is a tool to help you tap into your body's wisdom beyond just the basics of health and fitness.

Why Somatic Exercises Matter

In the main book, I shared the importance of somatic exercises. They're not like a typical workout. They are about listening closely to your body, letting go of tension, and moving in ways that feel liberating.

This Workbook is here to guide you through that process. It includes exercises, reflections, and space for your own notes. Whether you're just getting started or looking to deepen your practice, there's something in here for you.

The Benefits

- Enhanced Body Awareness: Get to know the subtle signals your body sends you.

- Stress Relief: Find your own ways to relax and unwind through movement.

- Improved Mobility: Enjoy moving more freely without the usual aches or stiffness.

- Emotional Balance: Explore how connecting with your body can help manage emotions.

- Mindfulness: Learn to appreciate the present moment more fully.

Encouragement

Approach this Workbook with curiosity and an open mind. It's meant to be a resource for you, and much of it will be created by you through you're own writing and notes. There's no one-size-fits-all here; your experience will be determined by what resonates with you personally.

Thank you for allowing me to guide you. I hope this work can bring you insight, joy, and a deeper connection with yourself.

With love,

Rose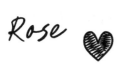

BODY SCAN

In Chapter 2, you read about how a strong mind-body connection can help you respond effectively to signals from your body. However, regulating a dysregulated nervous system can be hard when we don't take the time to hear what our body's signals mean.

So, as we perform our somatic exercise, we can do a simple body scan so that we're paying attention to the areas that come to our awareness. We can identify the feelings that come from the various parts of our body and then choose how we may respond to these feelings in a soothing way rather than trying to escape or ignore them.

Below, you will see a diagram of a body. Let's say that it's yours. Perform each exercise as guided by the book. Then, when you're ready, using the body diagrams below, take a pen and circle those parts of your body that emit a feeling that catches your attention. Draw a line from that part of your body to one of the boxes to the side, and use that space to answer the 3 questions shown below.

1. How did you feel before the exercise?

2. Did you experience any discomfort or aggravation during the exercise?

3. What feelings or emotions are you experiencing now the exercise is complete?

There are several repeats of this diagram so you can perform this activity multiple times. You'll be encouraged to do it again in Chapter 6.

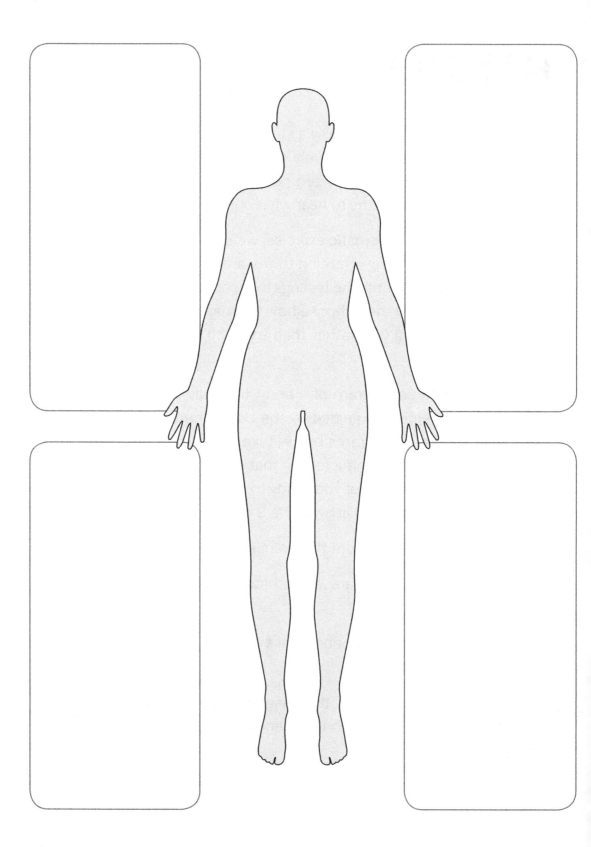

LearnWell, Somatic Exercises WORKBOOK

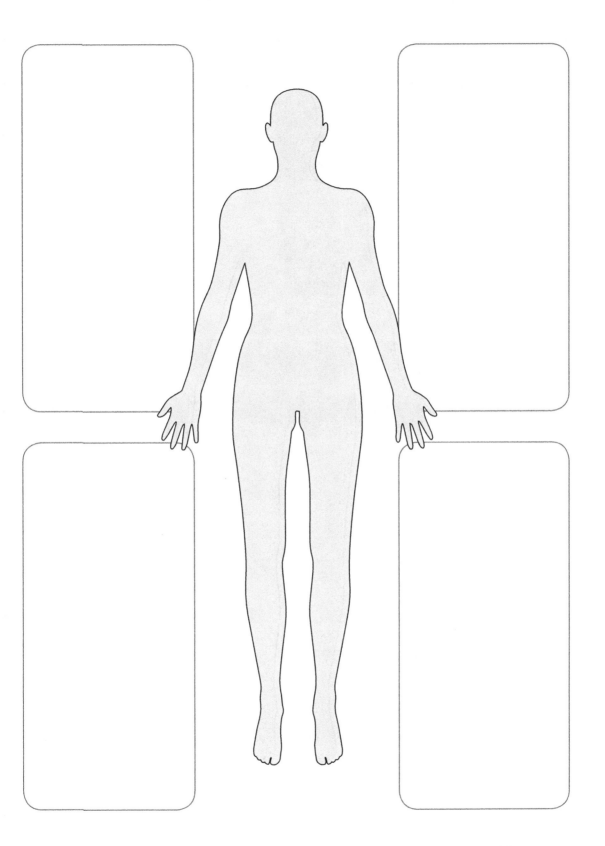

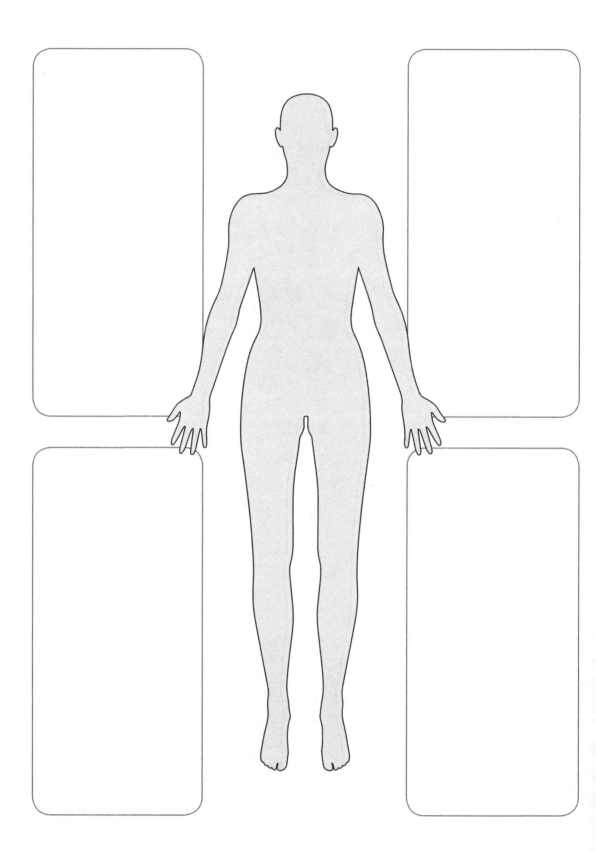

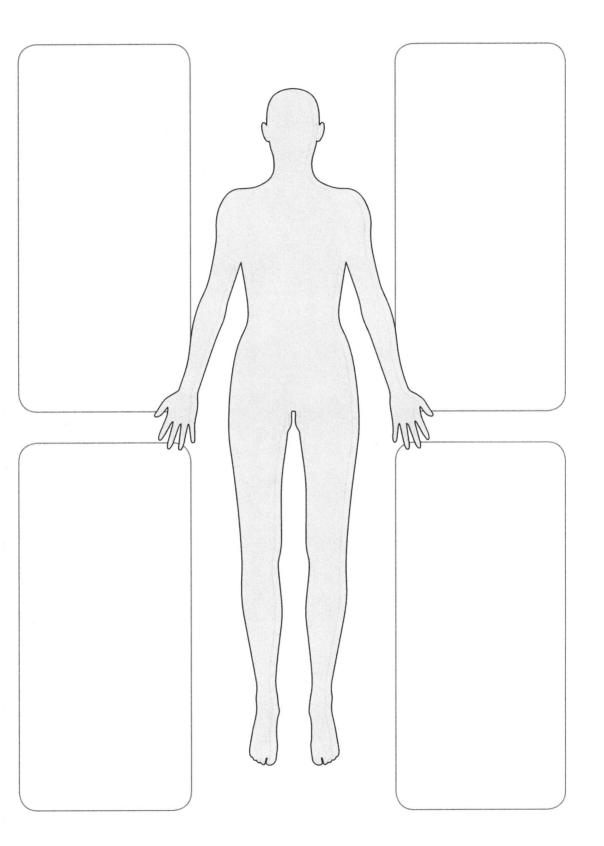

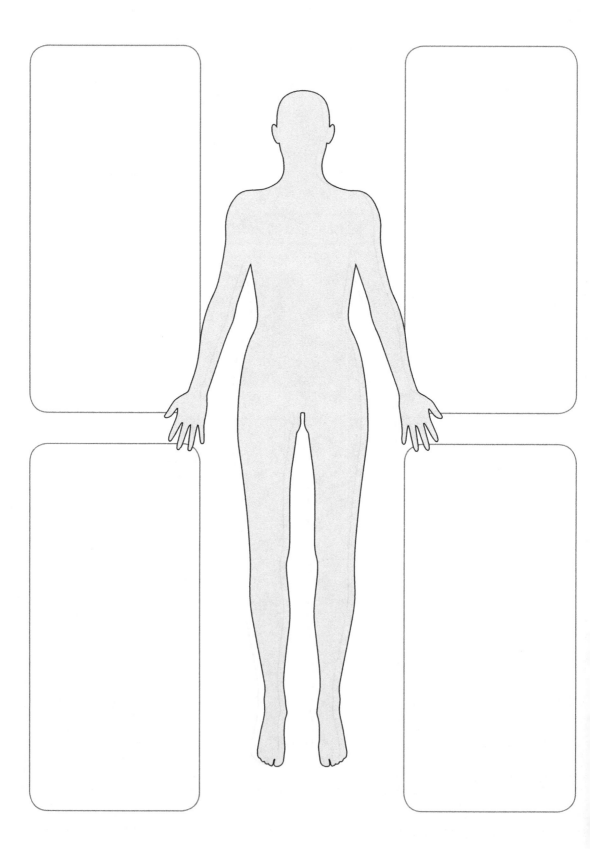

LearnWell, Somatic Exercises WORKBOOK

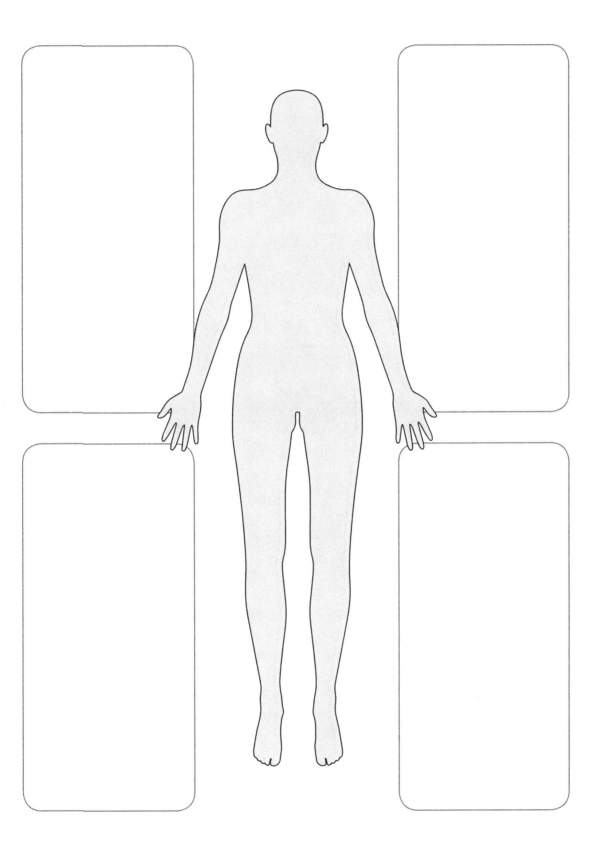

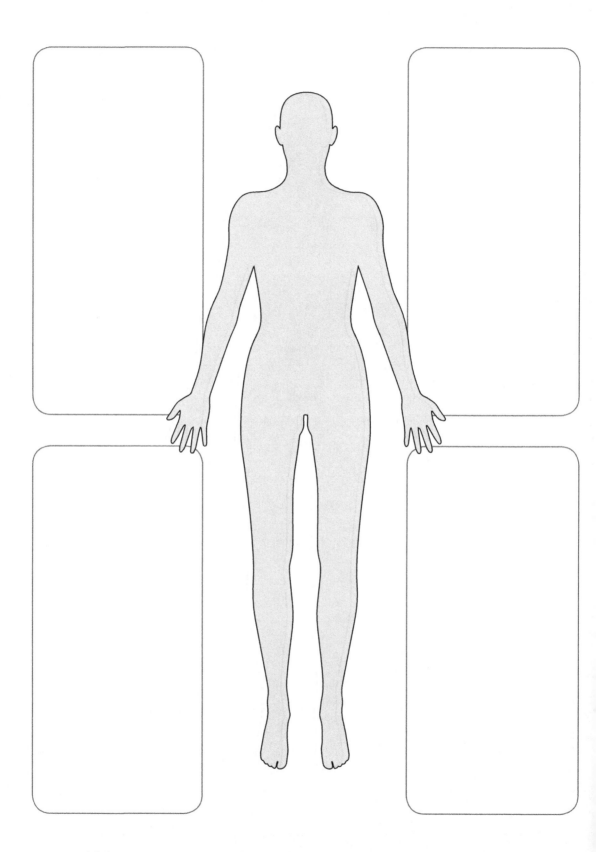

LearnWell, Somatic Exercises WORKBOOK

JOURNALING

You'll recall that I mentioned the concept of Somatic Journaling in the book. Here are the pages for a week of journaling to help you track your progress.

Keeping track of your progress is also a great way to know when you need to change things. If you follow your somatic exercise plan and don't see results for some time, it might be a sign that you're not feeling challenged enough.

This is an opportunity to reevaluate your daily 10-minute workout strategy. Maybe there's an exercise that you could switch out or deepen. Give yourself the benefit of the doubt and try out exercises you previously felt were out of your comfort zone.

Date: _____

Today I feel _____

Be open, vulnerable and expressive. Doing this enhances your mind-body awareness by creating an ability to acknowledge the feelings that your body is experiencing and trying to bring to your attention.

....

....

....

Today I performed these exercises ...

☐ ....

☐ ....

☐ ....

☐ ....

☐ ....

☐ ....

☐ ....

☐ ....

☐ ....

Following the exercises, I felt ...

....

....

....

I made physical progress in the following areas ...

....

....

....

My awareness has increased in the following areas ...

....

....

....

I achieved these goals in my practice today

....

....

....

Date: _____

Today I feel _____

Be open, vulnerable and expressive. Doing this enhances your mind-body awareness by creating an ability to acknowledge the feelings that your body is experiencing and trying to bring to your attention.

....

....

....

Today I performed these exercises ...

☐ ....

☐ ....

☐ ....

☐ ....

☐ ....

☐ ....

☐ ....

☐ ....

☐ ....

☐ ....

Following the exercises, I felt ...

....

....

....

I made physical progress in the following areas ...

....

....

....

My awareness has increased in the following areas ...

....

....

....

I achieved these goals in my practice today

....

....

....

Date: _____

Today I feel _____

Be open, vulnerable and expressive. Doing this enhances your mind-body awareness by creating an ability to acknowledge the feelings that your body is experiencing and trying to bring to your attention.

....

....

....

Today I performed these exercises ...

- [ ] ....
- [ ] ....
- [ ] ....
- [ ] ....
- [ ] ....
- [ ] ....
- [ ] ....
- [ ] ....
- [ ] ....
- [ ] ....

Following the exercises, I felt ...

....

....

....

I made physical progress in the following areas ...

....

....

....

My awareness has increased in the following areas ...

....

....

....

I achieved these goals in my practice today

....

....

....

Date: _____

Today I feel _____

Be open, vulnerable and expressive. Doing this enhances your mind-body awareness by creating an ability to acknowledge the feelings that your body is experiencing and trying to bring to your attention.

....

....

....

Today I performed these exercises ...

☐ ....

☐ ....

☐ ....

☐ ....

☐ ....

☐ ....

☐ ....

☐ ....

☐ ....

☐ ....

Following the exercises, I felt ...

....

....

....

I made physical progress in the following areas ...

....

....

....

My awareness has increased in the following areas ...

....

....

....

I achieved these goals in my practice today

....

....

....

Date: _____

Today I feel _____

Be open, vulnerable and expressive. Doing this enhances your mind-body awareness by creating an ability to acknowledge the feelings that your body is experiencing and trying to bring to your attention.

....

....

....

Today I performed these exercises ...

☐ ....

☐ ....

☐ ....

☐ ....

☐ ....

☐ ....

☐ ....

☐ ....

☐ ....

Following the exercises, I felt ...

....

....

....

I made physical progress in the following areas ...

....

....

....

My awareness has increased in the following areas ...

....

....

....

I achieved these goals in my practice today

....

....

....

Date: _____

Today I feel _____

Be open, vulnerable and expressive. Doing this enhances your mind-body awareness by creating an ability to acknowledge the feelings that your body is experiencing and trying to bring to your attention.

....

....

....

Today I performed these exercises ...

☐ ....

☐ ....

☐ ....

☐ ....

☐ ....

☐ ....

☐ ....

☐ ....

☐ ....

☐ ....

Following the exercises, I felt ...

....

....

....

I made physical progress in the following areas ...

....

....

....

My awareness has increased in the following areas ...

....

....

....

I achieved these goals in my practice today

....

....

....

Date: _____

Today I feel _____

Be open, vulnerable and expressive. Doing this enhances your mind-body awareness by creating an ability to acknowledge the feelings that your body is experiencing and trying to bring to your attention.

....

....

....

Today I performed these exercises ...

☐ ....

☐ ....

☐ ....

☐ ....

☐ ....

☐ ....

☐ ....

☐ ....

☐ ....

Following the exercises, I felt ...

....

....

....

I made physical progress in the following areas ...

....

....

....

My awareness has increased in the following areas ...

....

....

....

I achieved these goals in my practice today

....

....

....

QUESTIONNAIRE

As you prepare to build your exercise plan, it will help you to be mentally ready, as well as physically. I've prepared some questions below that will guide your mind to develop clear thoughts about your body's requirements.

Please go through the process. It will make a significant difference in the way you approach your exercises. Instead of just going through the motions, this will help you to truly connect with the benefit that each exercise brings to you, specifically.

Noticing Body and Emotional States

Observation of Sensations: What specific sensations do you notice in different parts of your body throughout the day (e.g., tension, relaxation, discomfort)?

....

....

....

Emotion-Body Connection: Can you link these sensations to particular emotions or states of mind you are experiencing?

....

....

....

Sensation Patterns: Are there recurring sensations in specific body parts associated with certain emotional experiences?

....

....

....

Identifying Areas for Attention

Frequent Sensation Locations: Which areas of your body frequently experience sensations, and what types of sensations are they (e.g., shoulders - tension, stomach - butterflies)?

....

....

....

Intensity and Duration: How intense and lasting are these sensations? Do they quickly pass, or are they persistent?

....

....

....

Physical Responses to Daily Events: How do different parts of your body respond to daily events, both positive and negative?

....

....

....

Emotional States and Physical Sensations

Comfort vs. Discomfort: In what areas of your body do you feel comfort or discomfort during various emotional states (e.g., "When I'm proud of myself, I feel X. When I'm anxious, I feel Y ...")?

....

....

....

Changes Over Time: Have you noticed any changes in where and how your body experiences these sensations over time?

....

....

....

Predictive Sensations: Are there physical sensations that predict certain emotional states or reactions from you?

....

....

....

Guiding Towards Somatic Exercises

Somatic Curiosity: Considering the sensations and areas you've identified, which of the somatic exercises are you most curious about or feel might be beneficial?

....

....

....

Attention and Care: Which parts of your body do you feel are asking for more attention and care based on your responses?

....

....

....

GOAL SETTING

Now that you're clearer on your unique and targeted needs, the next step toward a complete 10-minute somatic exercise plan is to set goals. There is space below to write down your goals.

Some tips to help you define clear and achievable objectives include:

- Be specific and clear.

- Choose measurable benchmarks.

- Have realistic expectations.

- Assign a realistic time frame to each goal.

- Ensure they align with your overall well-being.

- Be open to adjusting them if necessary.

- Celebrate your successes, no matter how small.

Take a moment to write your goals. Choose 2 easily attainable goals, 2 more challenging goals, and 1 main goal or objective.

Easy

....

....

....

....

Challenging

....

....

....

....

My main, overall goal

....

....

....

....

EXERCISE CHECKLIST

Below, you'll see a checklist of the 35 exercises you learned in Chapter 5. To build your daily plan, consider choosing up to 10 exercises on the list.

Depending on your overall goal and target areas, you can choose exercises from each section or fine-tune your selection to just one or two sections. If you're unsure, take some time to go back to Chapter 5 and feel which exercises are right for you.

They've been arranged below in 7 lists so that you can create a plan for a week. This ties in with the journaling and body scan exercises that you've read about above.

Make this checklist part of your Daily Plan. You'll read more about that below.

	DAY OF THE WEEK						

SECTION 1:
REVITALIZING THROUGH BREATH

Exercise 1: Diaphragmatic Breathing ☐ ☐ ☐ ☐ ☐ ☐ ☐

Exercise 2: Somatic Sighing ☐ ☐ ☐ ☐ ☐ ☐ ☐

Exercise 3: Somatic Breath Counting ☐ ☐ ☐ ☐ ☐ ☐ ☐

Exercise 4: Humming ☐ ☐ ☐ ☐ ☐ ☐ ☐

SECTION 2:
STRESS AND TENSION RELEASE

Exercise 5: Progressive Muscle Relaxation ☐ ☐ ☐ ☐ ☐ ☐ ☐

Exercise 6: Body Scan Meditation ☐ ☐ ☐ ☐ ☐ ☐ ☐

Exercise 7: Palm Pushing ☐ ☐ ☐ ☐ ☐ ☐ ☐

Exercise 8: Leg Shaking ☐ ☐ ☐ ☐ ☐ ☐ ☐

Exercise 9: Trauma-Releasing Exercises (Tre) ☐ ☐ ☐ ☐ ☐ ☐ ☐

Exercise 10: Somatic Writing ☐ ☐ ☐ ☐ ☐ ☐ ☐

Exercise 11: Guided Imagery ☐ ☐ ☐ ☐ ☐ ☐ ☐

SECTION 3:
SPINAL AND POSTURAL HEALTH

Exercise 12: Pelvic Tilts ☐ ☐ ☐ ☐ ☐ ☐ ☐

Exercise 13: Spinal Twists ☐ ☐ ☐ ☐ ☐ ☐ ☐

Exercise 14: Cat-Cow Stretch ☐ ☐ ☐ ☐ ☐ ☐ ☐

Exercise 15: Rolling Down The Spine ☐ ☐ ☐ ☐ ☐ ☐ ☐

Exercise 16: Child's Pose ☐ ☐ ☐ ☐ ☐ ☐ ☐

Exercise 17: Seated Forward Bend ☐ ☐ ☐ ☐ ☐ ☐ ☐

Exercise 18: Standing Forward Bend ☐ ☐ ☐ ☐ ☐ ☐ ☐

SECTION 4:
MINDFULNESS AND GROUNDING

Exercise 19: Grounding Exercises

Exercise 20: Mindful Walking

Exercise 21: Eye Palming

Exercise 22: Somatic Visualization

Exercise 23: Yoga Sun Salutations

SECTION 5:
GRACEFUL MOVEMENTS FOR FLEXIBILITY

Exercise 24: Tai Chi Movements

Exercise 25: Butterfly Pose

Exercise 26: Cross-Crawl Exercise

Exercise 27: Arm Stretching And Releasing

Exercise 28: Side Bends

Exercise 29: Knee-To-Chest Stretch

Exercise 30: Figure-Eight Hip Movements

Exercise 31: Psoas Release Exercise

Exercise 32: Lateral Neck Stretch

Exercise 33: Self-Massage

SECTION 6:
BALANCE AND FOCUS

Exercise 34: Balancing On One Foot

Exercise 35: Somatic Empathy Exercise

DAILY PLAN

Your plan is probably taking shape by now. You may have chosen your ten exercises and you're ready to start.

I've repeated a section from the book as a suggestion for how you may craft your own plan. However, your plan is, as it says - your own. So read below but then use the space below that to set out the way you'll perform your own exercises.

- 1-minute warm-up: One exercise to center the mind (ie. Somatic breath counting).

- 6 minutes of main exercises: this could be 3 exercises of your choice (2 minutes each).

- 2-minute release: A releasing exercise (ie. shaking or releasing visualization).

- 1-minute cool-down: One final exercise to process and integrate the experience (ie. Diaphragmatic breathing).

MY DAILY PLAN

I'm looking forward to performing the following exercises ...

DAY 1

MINS	EXERCISES
1	
2	
3	
4	
5	
6	
7	
8	
9	
10	

DAY 2

MINS	EXERCISES
1	
2	
3	
4	
5	
6	
7	
8	
9	
10	

DAY 3

MINS	EXERCISES
1	
2	
3	
4	
5	
6	
7	
8	
9	
10	

DAY 4

MINS	EXERCISES
1	
2	
3	
4	
5	
6	
7	
8	
9	
10	

DAY 5

MINS	EXERCISES
1	
2	
3	
4	
5	
6	
7	
8	
9	
10	

DAY 6

MINS	EXERCISES
1	
2	
3	
4	
5	
6	
7	
8	
9	
10	

DAY 7

MINS	EXERCISES
1	
2	
3	
4	
5	
6	
7	
8	
9	
10	

Thank you for allowing me to guide your practice. I sincerely hope you feel enormous benefit from your exercises. You deserve to feel good.

Love Rose

SPACE FOR YOUR NOTES

LearnWell, Somatic Exercises WORKBOOK

NOTES

NOTES

BOOK 2

TOOLS TO REGULATE YOUR NERVOUS SYSTEM

Somatic, Cognitive & Lifestyle Techniques
To Create Calm, Relieve Stress & Reduce Anxiety

To Mum.

Your calm amidst raging seas is
the greatest strength I've known

BOOK 2 CONTENTS

Introduction — 181

1   Flooded With Calm — 184
Your Magical Nervous System And Its Battle Against Stress

2   Your Puppet Master And How It Runs Your Life — 197
How Your Autonomic Nervous System Manages Your Stress

3   Some Hurt That Can Last Forever — 207
How Trauma Can Affect Your Nervous System

4   How To 'Chill Out' Properly — 215
Mind-Body Techniques For Stress Reduction

5   Using Your Body As A Tool To Create Calm — 227
Exercise And Movement For Melting Away Stress

6   Food To Fuel Your Flow — 236
The Role Of Nutrition In Stress Reduction

7   Snooze Your Way To Peace — 247
Why Sleep Is The Ultimate Path To A Calmer Life

8   Stress And The Friend-Factor — 256
Your Social Circles Can Create Or Damage Your World

9   The Harmony Highway — 271
Your Vagus Nerve And Why It's So Spectacular!

10   Make It All Happen — 281
How You Can Use These Tools In Real Life

References — 293

WORKBOOK

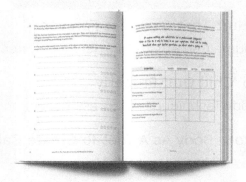

As you may have read earlier, to increase your retention of knowledge on this important topic, we have included a user-friendly Workbook that follows the content of this book, chapter by chapter. You will find the Workbook located on page 297. Alternatively, you can download and print a separate copy of the Workbook by following the link below:

Download A Copy Of The Workbook Here:

www.learnwellbooks.com/socalm

INTRODUCTION

Have you identified stress as a powerful force keeping you trapped? Are your stress and anxiety out of control, gradually leading you to breaking point?

Experiencing these symptoms can leave you in a desperate state, causing you to feel isolated from others and as though nobody understands what you're going through. Yet, you are far from alone. According to recent statistics, most Americans are experiencing extreme stress that affects mental health[1].

Before we discuss why that is the case, step back in time with me to 1995. It was when Alanis Morissette debuted in the music scene, releasing her first album, "Jagged Little Pill." I was in my mid-teens and an instant fan. Every time the song "Ironic" got airtime, I would drop everything to sing along with the lyrics.

The words appealed to my teenage mind in a *moth-to-the-flame* kind of way. I was adamant about soon stepping into an adult life of possibility, but this song depicted adult life in a manner I considered disappointing and somewhat shameful. I mean, the lyrics are murky with frustration and annoyance.

My "wise" teenage mind was conflicted about agreeing to adult life if this was it. I was just a teenager, and my only reference to adult life was from my observations about the carefree safety of being dependent. I was troubled by this image of the life I'd been looking forward to as it seemed like such a whirlpool of ironic incidents, leaving one stressed, weak, and tired.

Were adults blind to the secret of living a happy life? I was desperate to see what they were missing. All of this fueled my desire to avoid making the same mistakes previous generations were guilty of.

Now, decades later, my relentless search in this regard has changed my perspectives. I can say with absolute certainty that it is often not the lack of knowledge paralyzing our progress, causing frustration, stress, anxiety, and living a life robbed of joy and satisfaction. It is our lack of understanding of how to use our knowledge, bodies, and minds effectively is causing frustration, anxiety, and failure.

If people had a list of essential things they didn't quite understand but knew they needed to, the nervous system would be close to the top. This system is a powerful force, and the knowledge you have of this system, or the lack thereof, can enhance or limit your quality of life and expectations.

Understanding the nervous system's nature is the pivot between being oppressed by poorly managed stress and living a fulfilled life characterized by joy and satisfaction. Coupled with your ability to apply this knowledge to your advantage, it can empower you to excel in every area of life. But how can you make this breakthrough if the answers to your problems are so often shrouded in complex academic literature? When a mere attempt to grasp the content in a relevant matter does nothing but increase your stress levels? Or at least, that was the pickle I found myself in.

But once I understood the information I discovered during my in-depth studies on the nervous system and the body's response, I could identify the steps I had to take to manipulate this response to my advantage.

What I experienced and the improvements it brought to my life left me in awe, and I had to test my findings on others too. The more I shared my understanding of the nervous system and the steps I used to bring about change, the more I witnessed a transformation in the lives of others who followed my advice.

Chapter by chapter throughout this book, I share the same guidance with you. I do so in a manner that simplifies the complex academic terms. Instead of burdening you with academic material covering every physiological aspect of the nervous system, I extracted only the content relevant to the nervous system and your situation. I spoke about your need to better manage your stress.

The content I present in this book and its accompanying Workbook are practical guides to increase your understanding of effective ways to nurture this system. It offers advice on employing its full potential and setting yourself free. You'll gain a complete understanding of the nervous system, its nature, and how to apply it to enjoy optimal results.

The nervous system plays a leading role in your innate stress response, a response that naturally ripples out, affecting every aspect of your existence. If well-managed, it is a response that can empower you. But if you remain disempowered, allowing your nervous system to control you, it will keep you trapped, overwhelmed, and uncertain.

You can access the life you desire through advanced knowledge of the nervous system. This is a life of freedom, empowerment, calmness, fulfillment, and, most importantly, lasting happiness. The transformations I've seen over the past years in myself and others give me the confidence to promise that by following the practical steps in this book and the Workbook, you, too, can step into the life you desire.

But before we dig deeper into this process's practical steps, let's start by exploring the system itself. Then you'll realize that it is the most important tool to help you progress at the pace you're dreaming of and improve your overall well-being.

How long can you hang on before stress snaps the final cord keeping you connected to your sanity? This is your lifeline, your connection to an empowered, fulfilled life.

So, jump in and absorb every word of interest, idea, strategy, and technique from start to finish to benefit from this vital step toward freedom!

1

Don't forget to breathe

FLOODED WITH CALM

Your Magical Nervous System And Its Battle Against Stress

It is essential to have good tools, but it is also essential that the tools should be used in the right way.

– Wallace D. Wattles[2]

Your brain consists of roughly 100 billion nerve cells or neurons. Moving down the spine, you'll find another estimated 13.5 million of these cells[3]. Each neuron contributes to the total length of the system, estimated to be 37 miles![4]. The nervous system is delicately woven throughout the entire body, and through this complex network, life is possible. The nervous system controls life-sustaining actions, responses, and mental and emotional wellness. It plays a part in every aspect of your being. Being alive and the quality of life you experience depend on the nervous system. Yet, it often remains an underexplored aspect of human existence. Neglecting the care of this system, especially in the face of modern-day challenges, is at the heart of so many mental challenges and vulnerabilities people face today.

In the biological landscape beneath the skin, we stumble upon several mind-blowing systems complexly fused into each other. The nervous system stands out due to its immense control over the entire network. The puppetmaster controls every function and action, some of which you may be aware of, while others will slip by without notice. It ensures life-sustaining internal harmony and is essential in determining the quality of life. It is the one system impacting every aspect of your existence and demands not to be neglected.

WHAT IS THE NERVOUS SYSTEM?

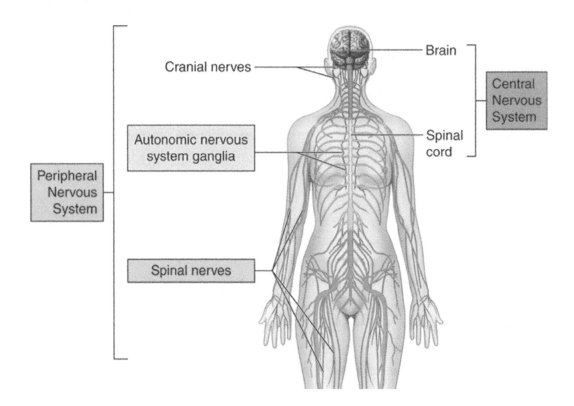

It would be impossible to explore this complex system without using new and rather scientific terminology, but understanding the nature of the nervous system is the key to propelling yourself toward the life you desire. So, let's dissect it into more easily understood parts. First, we can examine the central nervous system (CNS) and the peripheral nervous system (PNS).

THE CENTRAL NERVOUS SYSTEM

The CNS is the umbrella term referring to your brain and spinal cord. Both areas consist of compacted nerves covered in myelin (*mai-uh-lin*), the external layer protecting the nerve structure. It consists of protein and fat to insulate the nerves and ensure effective communication as impulses speed through your nerves, conveying vital messages to the relevant body parts. The CNS is the nervous system's headquarters, determining all bodily actions and responses, including intelligence, speech, the ability to feel, and the natural processes necessary to sustain life, like breathing.

THE PERIPHERAL NERVOUS SYSTEM

A more complex system to grasp is the PNS This system is the vast network of nerves branching out throughout the entire body, connecting HQ to the most remote areas, for example, the tips of your toes. It has two primary purposes; it collects information to feed to the CNS and conveys the message of how to respond from the CNS to various body parts.

Are you familiar with the excruciating pain caused by stepping barefoot on a Lego block at 2 am when all you wanted was a glass of water from the kitchen? This experience would not have been possible without the PNS. Failure of this system may not sound like a bad thing at 2 am, but the PNS is responsible for far more than merely conveying pain.

Feeling pain and reacting to it occurs in a part of the PNS known as the somatic nervous system. But it isn't the only role the PNS fulfills as it also consists of another section, the autonomic nervous system.

SOMATIC NERVOUS SYSTEM

The pain of stepping onto a Lego block, lifting your foot, pulling a painful face, and even withholding a scream of agony all occur with awareness. So, we can link sensations, responses, actions, or movements made with awareness, with the somatic nervous system. It is also responsible for all activities you want to do, like clapping your hands at your child's school play, texting your mother, or waving at a friend. You've *planned* these actions even though you may not know it was a planned move.

AUTONOMIC NERVOUS SYSTEM

The autonomic nervous system never enters the limelight as it manages all behind-the-scenes activities. Blood pressure, digestion, heart rate, and sexual arousal fall into the autonomic nervous system's portfolio. These are all life-sustaining actions occurring internally, even though you're unaware of them happening. Observing the autonomic nervous system in action requires more deliberate exploration, so it is quickly forgotten. But you'll soon notice when this system goes haywire. For example, when your blood pressure spikes, heart palpitations disrupt your peace, or a fading libido interferes with your love life. In this book, the autonomic nervous system is the main character at play. We'll explore various aspects of this system and how each part works together to ensure specific responses. Yet, even better, we'll explore how you can use multiple techniques to manipulate this system to your benefit. But first, I will break down this system into even smaller segments.

NEURONS – THE MOST ADVANCED BUILDING BLOCKS

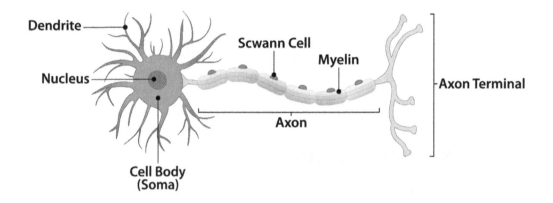

If we zoom in even further, the most basic units of the nervous system become visible. These are neurons. Neurons comprise a cell body with several antenna-like structures, or axons and dendrites, spiking from the nucleus's surface. Axons are usually long, untapered, and only branch out when they reach their target, while dendrites are short, tapered, and highly branched. These differences in structure between axons and dendrites are due to the different roles they fulfill. Dendrites are responsible for gathering information and must cover a large area to collect data and pass it to the cell body. Axons serve as messengers away from the cell body to another cell body or an organ.

These extensions give the neuron a spider-like appearance. Effective communication depends on healthy neurons as they are the building blocks in the communication network, conveying messages throughout the body.

HOW DOES IT WORK?

Well, what happened when you stepped on that Lego block? When you put your foot down on the block, the nervous system detects the sensation caused by the pressure of your weight on the block with the help of the dendrites and sends a message to HQ. The brain translates the feeling as pain and then relies on the axons to call every system throughout your body to deliver an appropriate response. It instructs the leg and foot muscles to lift your foot. Simultaneously it messages your facial muscles to express pain. Because it is 2 am, it makes a judgment call not to scream out in pain and refrains from instructing your vocal cords to exclaim in agony. This happens instantaneously and simultaneously and is only possible due to the complex system weaved throughout the entire body, the nervous system.

THE FUNCTIONS OF THE NERVOUS SYSTEM

This basic understanding of the nervous system's structure allows us to shift our focus to its functions. A deeper understanding of these functions provides an appreciation for the system in charge of your well-being before equipping yourself to create an optimal environment for your nervous system to flourish and improve your quality of life.

IT MAINTAINS AN OPTIMAL INTERNAL ENVIRONMENT

The nervous system manages the internal environment to ensure optimal health. One way it does this is by sweating. When you exercise or are physically active, your muscles build up heat. As the body needs to remain within a specific temperature window to prevent other devastating changes from occurring, the nervous system steps in to cool the body down. It sends messages to the blood vessels to expand, increasing blood flow to the skin to cool down on the surface. It also triggers increased sweating, using evaporation from the skin to cool down the body. And that is one of many ways it protects the perfect internal environment.

It Ensures Learning And Memory

You can thank your nervous system for everything you know, as it plays a vital role in learning and memory. Repeated actions turn new information into familiar knowledge. You've experienced this process countless times, like when learning to walk as a baby or writing your name when you're older.

It Enables Movement

Don't forget that the nervous system is the center from where every move you make is orchestrated. Jogging, walking, dancing, swimming, ice skating, or any other movement is possible because your nervous system controls every muscle to contract and relax at the right moment.

IT OFFERS PROTECTION

It keeps you safe. For deep thinking, areas in your brain will light up as they become active. But when your life depends on a sudden reaction, impulses are sent to the spinal cord, where a reflex reaction will get you to react in time to prevent injury. Pulling your hand from a hot surface before you sustain third-degree burn wounds, muscles contracting when you twist your ankle, preventing a fracture, or sneezing when something irritates your nose all fall into this category.

From underneath the umbrella of protection, we can extract the stress response. This response can save your life. Yet, it will also harm your mental, physical, and emotional wellness if you remain in this state for too long.

WHAT IS THE STRESS RESPONSE?

If it weren't for the stress response, we likely wouldn't have survived as a species. Another widely known term for this is the fight or flight response. To offer you a vivid image indicating this response's valuable role in ensuring survival, we'll have to step back much further in history than 1995. Let's revert to many, many years ago, before civilization, when the homo genus species were living in caves and hunting for meals.

THE CAVEMAN'S HUNT

Shhh. We find ourselves in a dangerous place. While we're hiding out of sight, too many threats lurking everywhere for our modern minds to fathom, so it is better to remain quiet and only observe.

We're in the jungle. The surrounding foliage is dense, and beneath our feet is the dark and clammy soil, rich in nutrients, sustaining life in this unkind environment. Dim light breaks through the thick canopy above, and it is in this light that we can spot his every move.

His length is disguised as he is bent forward slightly. In the low light, we can see his arched back and one hand raised above his head, holding a spear, nothing but a handcrafted wood tool with a sharpened stone tied to the end. Every step he takes is done deliberately after careful consideration. The caveman is on the hunt.

Sweat is pearling on his forehead while his nostrils flare open, sniffing the air for the scent of friend or foe. It had been days since he had anything to eat, and the growling sounds from within got him to venture beyond the safety of his cave, turning to the belly of the jungle in search of prey. Yet, just as quickly, the hunter can become the hunted, so he must remain on high alert. His life depends on every move. Yet, he is unaware of the internal biological processes, for his nervous system controls his every movement.

He stops and turns his head toward the direction a sound came from. His heart is pounding in his chest. Every muscle in his body is tense; his eyes are fixated on a shadow in the distance. He is ready to attack. He jumps. His arm shoots forward with perfected power and placement.

It all happens instantly. The growl, attack, noise, grunt, victory for one and death for another. He pulls his spear from the chest of his prey, dripping blood on the saber-toothed animal, dethroned in its own territory, and now nothing but a meal to feast on.

We've witnessed a spectacular show of precision and power inspired by the need for survival. But what is even more impressive is what occurred internally. A symphony of stimuli and responses occurred inside the body, a physiological showcase of perfection performing the fight or flight response.

Our minds were too deeply immersed in what we've witnessed to notice the sheer perfection of the body's response to a threat. No, we have to return to our current time, when modern science and advanced technology opened the internal landscape and revealed the complexity of the stress response.

THE STRESS RESPONSE UNDER THE MICROSCOPE

Let's look at what has occurred in our caveman's body. The moment he set foot outside his cave's safety and into the jungle, he was exposed to a stressor. This triggered the amygdala (*uh-mig-duh-luh*), the area in the brain responsible for emotional processing, to alert the hypothalamus (*hai-poh-tha-luh-muhs*) of exposure to threats[5]. The hypothalamus acts as the command center in the brain and instructs the entire body to get ready to fight or flee.

Before proceeding, let's pause to understand the amygdala's and hypothalamus's nature and function.

FUNCTIONS OF THE AMYGDALA AND HYPOTHALAMUS

The amygdala is a small structure located in the brain's center. Its shape and size are often compared to that of an almond. Despite its size, it remains a complex area responsible for emotional management. It regulates feelings like anxiety, fear, and aggression but is also responsible for emotional memory. When the amygdala is triggered, it immediately responds by instigating an emotional reaction. In our example, we can only assume that the caveman is familiar with threats in the jungle and has prior experience of fear when stepping outside of the safety of the cave. As the center of emotional processing, the amygdala is the area first triggered when exposed to a situation posing a threat.

The hypothalamus is similar to the amygdala in size and also located near the brain's center, but this is where the similarities begin to taper. This part of the brain controls hormonal control and links the endocrine (*en-dow-krine*) or hormonal system and the nervous system. The endocrine system comprises a network of hormone-releasing glands distributed across the body. The hypothalamus controls the release of hormones to fulfill various functions to ensure the body remains optimal. Again, referring to our example, once the amygdala alerts the hypothalamus, it will release stress hormones, like adrenaline and cortisol, to initiate the stress response to protect the caveman. But, as we'll see later, it is also responsible for releasing hormones to restore peace and calm within.

The nervous system uses these hormones to instruct the lungs to level up by breathing faster. It also causes the smallest bronchioles to open up to allow higher oxygen uptake and ensure a more effective oxygen transfer to the blood. These changes provide sufficient oxygen in the muscles to fight or flee quickly. Extra oxygen also travels to the brain, keeping it on high alert.

Changes in the arteries and veins ensure higher blood pressure, guaranteeing better distribution of oxygen and nutrients. It also means that circulation is reduced towards systems that aren't playing a part in the fight or flight response. I am specifically thinking about the digestive, reproductive, and immune systems.

As all of these processes cause the body's heat to increase, sweat glands are activated to cool down the skin's surface to manage the body's temperature.

Eyes are dilated so that the caveman can observe his environment better to become aware of the threat or any attack quickly. As the body is ready for action, you may notice that there is a bit of a tremble in his muscles. This isn't fear, as we so popularly like to believe. No, this indicates the body's readiness for anything that may come its way.

What a magnificent response this is, indeed! One trigger is enough to set off the nervous system to prepare the body and brain for anything coming. It kept the caveman safe, enabling him to fight or run away fast.

Let's be clear. This process is a good thing ... if you're exposed to an actual threat. Yes, exposure to a real danger means that your body is spending only a limited time in this state of high stress. Once the caveman in our story planted his spear into his prey's chest, the nervous system signaled that the threat was over and all could return to normal. His heart rate slowed, breathing returned to normal, and so did all the other changes due to this response.

WHEN GOOD TURNS TO BAD – AND WHY IT HAPPENS

In the current day and time, we don't hunt for food any longer. The concrete urban jungle is the only jungle most people have ever encountered. Yet, we still face many stressors that trigger the same physiological response. These stressors come in the form of broken relationships, lay-offs at work, the trauma of being mugged, a bleak economic environment, deadlines, and the many uncertainties the future holds.

Exposure to these triggers brings the same stress response in the body. But these threats don't quickly disappear. The body engages in the same stress response, and this state can remain present for days, weeks, months, or even longer.

While the human body can deal with high-stress conditions for short stints, it faces a complete breakdown if exposure is prolonged. For example, your body is well-equipped for the stress response when running away from danger. But today, the stress response is more often triggered by threats like financial strain. This is a stressor against which you can't defend yourself with physical activity. It is also a stressor remaining present and putting the body in a high-stress state for longer. If this is the case, we look at an entirely different outcome in the body.

Prolonged exposure to the stress response weakens the system, causing health concerns.

This is a key concept to appreciate

- Chronic high blood pressure leads to heart health challenges, heart attacks, and strokes.

- The immune system remains neglected, resulting in the body getting sick more often.

- The digestive system suffers the same continued neglect, deteriorating and causing problems like indigestion, constipation, diarrhea, diabetes, and obesity.

- Cholesterol levels spike.

- Breathing problems occur, and the body may develop asthma.

- These symptoms, caused by prolonged exposure to the fight or flight state, lead to chronic fatigue, headaches, migraines, and even sexual dysfunction.

- This wave of negative consequences spreads wide, affecting mental health too. Persistent high-stress levels lead to anxiety, depression, panic disorders, and other mental health concerns. **???**

Where do you find yourself in all of this? Are you at the shortest end of the stick? The one whose body is gradually breaking down under the pressure of prolonged exposure to the stress of the fight or flight response?

WHERE DOES THIS LEAVE YOU?

When I first came to understand the complexity of the stress response, I was experiencing two conflicting emotions. Of course, I was in extreme awe at how amazing the mind and body collaborate, but a sense of helplessness surfaced.

In my mind, a shrieking voice asked many questions. *Am I a victim of my nervous system's response? Where is my voice in all of this? Can I even take control of my body's response to a breakup, financial stress, or any of life's many stressors?*

The good news is that while you can't restrict your life to the extent that you're never exposed to stressors—that wouldn't even constitute living—you can manage it. We'll explore many holistic techniques to care for the mind, body, and soul, including your nervous system. It is how you can take control of your life. Through these steps, you can prevent dire mental and physical health concerns caused by a system that lost direction in an ever-changing modern environment. A system so powerful it can easily transition from protector to threat.

 Spend a moment now to explore your Workbook. You'll enjoy the journaling activity and the thoughtful exercises that relate specifically to your own life.

When you're ready to explore more about this vital system, a system that is behind almost every sensation and emotion you feel right now, a system that most likely is behind the mood you're in, join me in the next chapter. There we'll go into the detail of even smaller segments of the nervous system and extend our gaze from how it causes your stressed state to how you can use it to enter a state of relaxation.

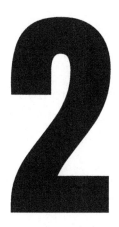

YOUR PUPPET MASTER AND HOW IT RUNS YOUR LIFE

How Your Autonomic Nervous System Manages Your Stress

Take a deep breath... Inhale peace.
Exhale happiness.

– A.D. Posey[5]

Let's go to the jungle! There is more to learn from our caveman.

We're back, surrounded by luscious green jungle plants. Each of them competes for sunlight, mere fragments of light scattered on the damp soil of the forest floor. Only a few rays break through the dense canopy above, leaving a musty smell in the air, a scent familiar to the caveman.

With a grunt, the caveman expresses his satisfaction while wiping his spear clean on the prey's fur, and a sweet sense of victory fills the air.

This image, the brute force of the kill, is light years removed from your clean, organized, and highly automated existence, right? Or is it? Perhaps modern society isn't so different.

When we strip away everything that sets us apart from him, the realization sinks in that underneath the skin, the same driving forces control life.

MEET KIM

Kim is in her early fifties, a successful entrepreneur who has made overzealous business decisions over recent months, putting her business, a medium-sized marketing agency, in a vulnerable position. While Kim tried to keep the reality of her enterprise's financial health under the covers, a disgruntled employee seized the moment to blurt her secrets to the competition. Now, Kim is facing a stand-off in her own office.

Can she protect her reputation, key clients, and trusted employees from her competitors poised to swoop in on her misfortune? They are sitting across from her at her boardroom table, discussing the terms of a hostile takeover, poorly disguised as a merger. Or will she secure lifesaving financial support from third-party investors that will allow her to fight another day in this brutally competitive industry?

Kim's body responds in the exact same manner as the caveman's did. Her pupils are dilated as she is looking the enemy in the eye. Her powerful deodorant hides excessive sweating while her soaked armpits are hidden within her armor, a power suit, the most elegant in corporate wear. Yet, it is much harder to hide the pearls of sweat forming on her forehead. Her breathing is shallow, and her movements are slow and precise. She is buying herself time. She is waiting for a call before she pens her name to paper.

There is a knock at the door before it's flung open. She looks up. Her secretary is there in a superhero's stance but without a cape. The secretary gives the nod, a sly grin, and with that, Kim tears up the paperwork on her desk in a gesture of victory. With relief, she marches her competitors out the front door and slams it behind them as they leave. She got the funding she needed and saved her firm in the nick of time.

Her thumping heart starts to slow down, her blood pressure eases, and she joins her secretary in a celebratory lunch. Her appetite was restored as blood circulation returned to normal, and hunger reminded her that she hardly ate for days.

Whether we're looking at the life of the caveman or the modern-day person, there are many undeniable resemblances. Yes, the autonomous system is still in charge, but what sets civilization apart is our insight into physiology through modern science. These advances offer a deeper understanding of the complex systems controlling life and serve as a gateway to guide us to utilize these systems, like the nervous system, to our benefit.

GAINING BENEFITS THROUGH INSIGHT INTO THE STRESS RESPONSE

In this chapter, we explore what happened in Kim's and the caveman's bodies and minds from the moment they overcame the cause of their stress as they made the deal or the kill. They walked away with relief and satisfaction with their respective outcomes. Their blood pressure drops as their heart rate slows down. Circulation returns to normal, supplying blood to the digestive, immune, and reproductive systems. Underneath their skins is a different symphony of processes working together to ensure their happiness, satisfaction, and relaxation, a state of optimal well-being.

These symphonies of internal systems are controlled by one single force. The autonomic nervous system is the conductor at the helm of this response, returning the body to a state of calm and restoring inner harmony effortlessly. A deeper understanding of the autonomic nervous system and how it orchestrates calm makes it possible to manually manipulate these systems to restore internal calm amidst stressful factors.

In the previous chapter, I touched on the autonomic nervous system, which is part of the PNS, but there is much more to say. When we place the autonomic nervous system under the microscope, an entire world of possibilities opens up. It is a world heavy with opportunities to utilize this system to your benefit by controlling your state of mind and, therefore, your mental, physical, and emotional states.

DIVIDING THE AUTONOMIC NERVOUS SYSTEM INTO SMALLER DIVISIONS

We can divide the autonomic nervous system into three smaller distinct divisions. These are the sympathetic, parasympathetic, and enteric systems. The enteric system (ENS) fulfills roles like nutrient uptake, food peristalsis in the digestive system, and immune defense. To a certain extent, it also regulates blood. It plays a role in the stress response, but as it is mainly linked to the gut, a topic discussed in chapter six, I'm placing it on the side for now.

The two divisions we will focus on now are the sympathetic and parasympathetic systems.

The sympathetic nervous system (SNS) fulfills a key role during the stress response, while the parasympathetic nervous system (PSNS) is responsible for restoring a state of calm. To enjoy optimal lasting health and wellness, these two systems in a yin and yang relationship must be in complete harmony.

Remember this. It will appear several times.

TAKING A CLOSER LOOK AT THE SYMPATHETIC NERVOUS SYSTEM

The (SNS) originates in the spinal cord. It consists of a pathway of clusters of nerve fibers, or ganglia (*gang-glee-uh*). The ganglia in the SNS can be divided into three types based on the kind of nerve cells it consists of, which are preganglionic, sympathetic, and postganglionic. Each has unique features and functions[6].

While there is much detail to share about the different types of ganglia, it wouldn't contribute to our cause of determining how to achieve effective management and control of the nervous system to restore a state of calm in the face of adversity. Hence, we do not need to explore these fibers in greater detail.

What is crucial for us is to know that this system controls the stress response. Once it receives an impulse triggering the response, it prepares the entire body to undergo several changes. Some of the physical changes you can expect are your heart rate speeding up to ensure sufficient oxygen supply to various body parts. The pupils enlarge to allow more light in and so improve vision. It slows down the digestive tract to reduce the energy consumption in this area to secure sufficient energy supply to other places. It also relaxes the lung muscles, allowing more air and increasing the oxygen supply. At the same time, the liver is also involved in the process, releasing energy to supply the muscles with the fuel it needs to run faster or fight stronger. We've been through this process in the previous chapter, and there is nothing else to add. Hence, I am shifting your focus to the parasympathetic nervous system and the responsibilities it is tasked with to restore calm and inner peace.

THE PARASYMPATHETIC NERVOUS SYSTEM

The behavior of the caveman after the kill, and Kim's reactions after she shuts the door behind her competitors, reflect the parasympathetic nervous system (PSNS) in action. Once they could disengage from the looming threat, their PSNS was naturally triggered to restore calm in body and mind. For them, the relationship between these two systems worked perfectly and as it should under the right circumstances. The natural response in an ideal world would be a threat–SNS (Sympathetic)–

action–PSNS (Parasympathetic)–calm, but we don't live in an ideal world. No, modern-day threats don't have the same simplicity as the straightforward, even though very scary, threats found in the world of the caveman.

The primary purpose of the PSNS is to bring calm to the body and mind and to restore equilibrium in the internal landscape. Once triggered, it, too, orchestrates an entire symphony of functions and processes, even though it is a somewhat different showcase than what was delivered by the SNS. The performance of the PSNS wouldn't have been possible without the vagus nerve. The vagus nerve's role in the PSNS is so crucial that I dedicate an entire chapter focusing on it later. Yet, it is essential to understand the role the vagus nerve has to play and where it fits into the PSNS.

The vagus nerve is responsible for several functions regulating overall wellness like digestion, heart rate, specific reflex responses, and respiratory, but that isn't all. It also plays a role in stress management as part of the PSNS, making up about 75% of the PSNS. Its key responsibility in this regard is to gather information from the organs and convey it to the brain. Based on its structure, we can say that the vagus nerve is the link in the brain-gut axis (something I'll expand on in chapter six). However, it is also responsible for triggering several of the reactions listed below as part of the physiological response restoring a state of inner calm[7].

Let's overview the various processes the mind and body rely on to restore calm.

- The pupils constrict, limiting the amount of light penetrating the eyes. This improves close-up vision and increases the production of tears to sustain healthy eyes.

- The lung muscles contract, reducing the work necessary for breathing during resting periods.

- Heart rate slows down, and blood pressure reduces.

- Circulation returns to the digestive, immune, and reproductive systems.

- The digestion system also triggers the pancreas to release more insulin to break down sugar.

- Saliva glands in the nose and mouth increase saliva production, as this helps with breathing and digestion.

- The waste removal system relaxes to make urination and defecation possible.

While the body enters a state of relaxation, so does the mind. You'll feel relaxed and calm, entering a mental, emotional, and physical state characterized by positivity.

Can you see that both systems are vital for sustained harmony and protection?

For the caveman, switching from one system to another happened organically. But the same is no longer true for us in modern society. The threats we face originate differently. By nature, they don't resolve once physical action is taken. The result is much more prolonged exposure to high-stress states and remaining in control of the SNS longer than the body's ability to manage. While the body is well equipped to be in a state caused by the SNS, it can't remain here long. If exposure to the conditions of this state is too long-lasting, a range of physical and mental health concerns step in. It turns a system designed to protect you into a threat to your well-being.

But all isn't lost. Modern technology offers a deeper insight into what takes place internally. This knowledge enabled experts to unveil several techniques for manually flipping the switch, taking control from the SNS and handing it to the PSNS, restoring inner equilibrium.

YOU CAN FLIP THE SWITCH—TAKING YOUR BODY FROM SNS TO PSNS

You don't have to remain high-stress for longer than necessary. I am discussing many steps you can add to your collection of remedies to ensure effective stress management. The following is an overview of what you can expect to explore more thoroughly. Each step I list below holds the potential to bring you the relief and control you desire, the freedom to feel peace even when facing life's challenges. They are all steps helping you gain power and control in this transition to manually direct your nervous system, instigating a calm state in your mind and body. They promise instant results and will relieve your immediate concerns.

MASSAGE

Even a short session with a qualified and experienced masseuse can bring your mind peace and your body calm on all levels. A massage is a solution that will bring instant relief, but with repeated sessions, you can also establish lasting improvement. There are plenty of benefits to reap from regular sessions. Massaging can retrain your body to transition from an SNS state to a PSNS state of relaxation. Gradually, it will become easier to switch naturally as your body regains familiarity with its inherent abilities.

MEDITATE

Separating yourself from stress or avoiding stressful factors or situations may not be on the cards for you, but this doesn't remove you from having control over your situation. While you may never have complete autonomy over your external environment, you have the power to manage internal stress effectively. Meditation plays a vital role in improving your natural response to external stressors. It helps the mind to reduce internal chatter and so contributes to calming down emotions. During meditation, the heart rate slows down, and so does breathing. Furthermore, the ancient practice helps to lower blood pressure and even contributes to healing by minimizing the amount of lactic acid trapped in the muscles.

Meditation may appear to be a mental process. However, success in meditation still depends on how effectively you can use your breathing to initiate a state of psychological and physical relaxation.

YOGA

Yoga has a slightly different approach than meditation, but in many ways benefits the mind and body in the same manner. It also serves to retrain the mind to transition between SNS and PSNS more naturally and without delay.

EXERCISE

When you opt for intensive exercises, you will likely trigger an SNS response, but light cardio, like a brisk walk, has the opposite effect. Are you familiar with the sense of calm flowing over you when you go for a walk after exposure to a stressful situation? The calm and relaxing experience you have is the PSNS system in action, a process activated by your level of physical activity.

SLEEP MORE

This one can be tricky as you may already find it hard to get the necessary shut-eye your body needs when constantly stressed. Still, when you get a proper amount of sleep, your body is far more prone to enter a state of PSNS with much greater ease.

BREATH WORK

Later, in chapter nine, we're placing the work of the vagus nerve under the microscope. The functions of this nerve are closely linked to breathing, and you'll learn how to use your breath to lower your stress levels. For now, let's hang onto the knowledge that you can transition your state of being by taking a few deep, slow breaths. This is likely the simplest way to reduce your stress instantly.

Are you ready to try it now?

- Breathe in slowly while counting to four.

- Hold your breath for four counts before slowly releasing the air while counting to four.

- Repeat the cycle 10 times and feel your body is changing from being in a state of high stress to much calmer.

These steps all have one thing in common—using the body to trigger the PSNS—ensuring calmness and relaxation. Through the mind-body connection, you can expect success when using any of these techniques to alter your mental state.

Before you continue, spend some time in your Workbook. Take a moment to breathe and contemplate the points in this chapter. More is to come; being relaxed will help you fully apply the knowledge I share.

THE POWER IS IN YOUR HANDS

Underestimating your power to manage your stress response will harm your health and wellness. It is why the remainder of the book predominantly focuses on various techniques guiding you to use your body and physical actions or activities to improve your state of mind.

Understanding this phenomenon—the mind-body connection—offers a science-based tool to utilize your body to improve your mental state and overall wellness. Know that the mind-body connection can easily slip into a negative loop too, but now is the time to change the order of things.

Before exploring the tools you have to improve your stress management and to bring you relief through the mind-body connection, we have to make one more pitstop to understand your current state. This stop takes us to the impact of trauma on the nervous system. Trauma is the type of exposure leaving a lasting impact on your life, scattering obstacles in your quest for deep relaxation. Traumatic exposure of any kind is a concern you must consider in your recovery, but knowing what you're up against provides you with the ideal platform to propel you toward success.

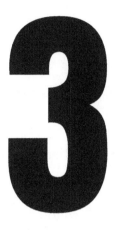

SOME HURT
THAT CAN
LAST FOREVER

How Trauma Can Affect
Your Nervous System

There are wounds that never show on the body that are deeper and more hurtful than anything that bleeds.

– Laurell K. Hamilton[8]

"I'm just going to grab a soda. Go on! I'll catch up with you!" Jake runs into the convenience store for refreshments while his friends continue down the street. They're 16, and the school holidays have just started. The youngsters are looking forward to their break, away from school, academics, and especially Mr. Dobson, their English Literature teacher. Jake opens the fridge door at the back of the store when he hears the man's voice in the front of the store.

"Shut up and just empty the cash register!" The man in the hoodie screams at the woman behind the counter.

She is old, and Jake can see her reflection when he quietly closes the fridge door. She looks upset. She is going to scream.

Jake can see her shaking. She started to cry and pleaded for her life. He sees how her hand reaches out to press a panic button.

'Don't. Don't. Don't.' The voice in his mind repeats the same mantra. 'Just give him the money,' his internal voice expands.

Jake finds himself paralyzed with fear. The wise thing should be to lie on the floor, but he can't even get himself to do that.

Then it happens.

She screams.

The shot.

"No! No!" the robber shouts. He grabs his bag and runs out.

Jake, still paralyzed, just stands in one spot. He can't move. Then he feels it. The warmth against his leg. He wet his pants.

His friends come running in. They heard the shot and saw the man running.

Chaos erupts around him, but Jake doesn't partake. His entire being is in shock.

"Is she dead?" is all that Jake could say.

Trauma takes many forms and can present itself in your life in numerous ways.

DEFINING TRAUMA AND ITS TYPES

Trauma results from experiencing a frightening, stressful, or distressing event or period of time.

There are certain types of trauma. If you've been exposed to any of these forms, you will likely carry remnants of this trauma with you for the rest of your life. As long as you don't address the effect trauma has on your life, it will impact your ability to manage your stress response well.

One of the most common types of trauma occurs on school grounds across the globe. Bullying is mostly associated with schools, but we can forget that bullying is also present in relationships and offices. Children or teenagers who bully often continue their behavior in adulthood, creating more victims by subjecting them to this type of trauma.

Community violence is a type of trauma that occurs when you're exposed to violence in the environment you stay in. You may not know the victim but are aware of the traumatic event and are duly aware of the dangers lurking on your streets the moment you step out of your home. It is a type of trauma often linked to witnessing warfare or even closer to home in dangerous neighborhoods riddled with crime on the streets.

Exposure to multiple traumatic events is called complex trauma and can significantly impact your life. This trauma includes childhood abuse, neglect, rejection, and witnessing domestic violence. While this sounds harsh, it is often the reality that if you're trapped in exposure to any of these mentioned crimes, you're likely a victim of several other types of traumatic experiences too.

Natural disasters like tornadoes, floods, and earthquakes can also constitute trauma. These events usually occur abruptly and can be devastating to experience as it is accompanied by the devastation and loss of loved ones and your safe environment.

Other severe examples of trauma are acts of terrorism, violence, sexual abuse, sex trafficking, or losing a loved one through abandonment or death.

THE EFFECT OF TRAUMA ON YOUR NERVOUS SYSTEM

While this isn't common, it has happened a few times to me. The first time it did, was many years ago when I just got my driver's permit. I was driving my dad's car, and being young and a bit of a show-off, I just had to pull over when I saw a friend walk next to the road. We chatted for a while before I decided to head home. My mind was in a million places and not behind the wheel. I did that day what I believe was the stupidest thing. I turned the key in the ignition, forgetting that throughout our conversation, the engine was idling the entire time.

The car made the most horrible noise, and I was instantly sure I just damaged my dad's car beyond repair. 'You're in so much trouble!' my mind convicted me over my negligence.

Well, thankfully it wasn't that bad, but I'll never forget the grinding sound of my mistake. As my knowledge of cars and engines evolved, I realized that if this were a regularly repeated mistake, there could be damage to various parts of the starter that would result in costly repairs. My dad's car was an older model with worn parts, so I had a lucky escape that day, and I didn't cause severe damage.

Exposure to trauma always reminds me of this day. Except for trauma having as much of a grinding effect on the body as the sound of that day had on my ears, it also poses the risk of causing lasting damage. Trauma equates to stress exposure interrupting your internal rhythm. It is like turning the key in the ignition too far for too long, seizing parts of the motor in a state of high stress.

Then the PNS loses its ability to regulate itself. If it gets stuck in this state, it becomes impossible to manage your emotions, and you'll remain in the fight or flight response. Staying in a physical state of hyperarousal is devastating to your physical and emotional health. Any attempt to gain control over your stress management will be futile until you address the impact of past trauma on your life.

If you're a victim like Jake and suffered from an acute traumatic incident, recovery can start soon after the incident, and there is no need to extend your suffering. But it is different if you experience complex trauma consisting of several types of traumatic events or chronic trauma, which is the long-term exposure to trauma in the past or present. Then, you'll have to free yourself first. Healing is impossible as long as you're exposed to the source of your trauma.

THE WINDOW OF TOLERANCE

To fully understand the impact of exposure to trauma, we must stand still at the window of tolerance for a while. Daily, you experience fluctuations in your nervous system. Exposure to a trigger activates the SNS, immersing your body in the stress response. As the threat passes, the PSNS kicks in, and you enter a calm state. This fluctuation is normal and occurs within the window of tolerance, where your emotional state may vary, but you can continue your daily activities.

Outside of this window is a state of hyper-arousal on one end and hypo-arousal on the other. The latter is the most extreme form of calm, characterized by numbness, shutting down, feeling ashamed, or even depression. On the opposing end of the spectrum is a state of hyper-arousal linked to the stress response. You'll find emotional overwhelm, racing thoughts, panic, and anxiety at this end.

Everyday stressful events will keep you safely within the window of tolerance. Still, when exposed to traumatic events, these events push you outside of the barriers of the window of tolerance. Which way you go varies from person to person, and you can either enter a state of hypo-arousal or hyper-arousal. For example, Jake froze, physically and emotionally, when he was confronted with trauma the day in the convenience store.

Being confronted by an armed man is something most people consider a threat. Yet, that said, everyone has a unique filtering system determining whether the situations they're confronted with are dangerous or a threat to them or not. These filters are set to protect you from reacting to every stimulus you're exposed to[9].

Once you've been pushed beyond the edges of the window of tolerance, these systems are damaged, and it becomes much harder to distinguish which events are a cause for concern for your safety and which aren't. Then even the most significant trigger can cause the SNS to react, putting you in the stress response. This is not a healthy state to remain in. You're losing the ability to distinguish between real threats and matters that aren't devastating. It results in complete dysregulation of the nervous system, causing changes to the neuron system. Initially, these changes are still reversible, but when there is persistent exposure to trauma, they become chronic and are at the core of post-traumatic stress disorder (PTSD)[9].

All isn't lost, though. You don't have to remain in this state of constant stress and nervous system deregulation, as several types of therapy have been proven to be highly successful in alleviating your challenges.

MIND-BODY APPROACHES TO OVERCOME PAST TRAUMA

Every strategy discussed in this book will provide valuable support to help you overcome the impact past trauma had on your life. Yet, trauma is a severe concern, and you'll most likely need professional therapy to address the challenges you're facing effectively.

Five types of therapy are popular in this regard as they are so effective.

COGNITIVE PROCESSING THERAPY

Cognitive processing therapy (CPT) is conducted by a mental health professional qualified in this field. The type of therapeutic treatment focuses on identifying irrational internal narratives or thoughts linked to the trauma you've experienced. For example, flood victims may fear the same event will happen even when a light drizzle is outside. Fearing a flood, in this case, is clearly irrational and linked to the trauma you've experienced during the flood. You'll identify these thoughts in therapy and practice new skills to reduce emotional dysregulation[9].

EYE MOVEMENT DESENSITIZATION AND REPROCESSING

EMDR or eye movement desensitization and reprocessing's primary focus is to unburden you of any negative emotional links to the traumatic event and to shift your focus to finding the positives that resulted from this event. Sometimes it is hard to see the silver lining around the dark cloud, but every event, even the ones which are so predominantly negative, has a positive outcome or element attached to it too. The relief patients in this therapy experience are significant, and EMDR is highly recommended to overcome trauma[9].

PROLONGED EXPOSURE THERAPY

During the initial traumatic moment, your mind and body are exposed to a certain extent of trauma. Still, your mind adds to the trauma afterward, and your memories can become more severe. Through prolonged exposure (PE) therapy, your therapist will help you to process these memories. Increased familiarity with these emotions reduces the overwhelming impact of your memories, and you'll realize that while the event was traumatic, you're no longer in danger[9].

SOMATIC EXPERIENCING

Somatic Experiencing (SE) was designed with a specific focus on helping trauma patients. The predominant focal points of this therapy are to identify and acknowledge your symptoms. Then you can draw on your resources and work to overcome these symptoms effectively. Once these memories no longer threaten you, you can revisit them without experiencing fear[9].

TALK THERAPIES

Specific talk therapies help you share your thoughts and feelings linked to the trauma you've experienced. These talk therapies are effective as they encourage you to revisit your memories and the events that caused you the trauma you experienced.

MOVEMENT PRACTICE

These are all highly effective manners to relieve yourself from the burden of trauma, but one more approach is gaining ground in this regard: movement practice. It is a type of therapy combining therapy and movement to release trauma from the body, and it is often taking on the form of yoga. It relies on deep breathing and yoga movements to activate the PSNS to restore a state of calm. For this, too, you'll need a trauma-informed yoga instructor to assist you.

It can be hard to imagine being free, while still trapped in trauma's grip and having it consume your life. The first vital step is creating physical distance between yourself and the cause of your traumatic exposure. Then, any of the mentioned therapy options can unlock mental freedom, taking you to complete recovery, as they'll help you to reset your stress response. Then the strategies I share will ensure effective stress management. This is management made possible through the mind-body connection, an inherent part of your being. Join me in the next chapter where we'll explore the first tool in your kit of stress management tools and how to master them to your benefit. Also, visit the Workbook to determine whether you're burdened by the impact of past trauma and are held back in a manner you're not even aware of.

In case you'd like to know more about this, LearnWell has produced a great book on healing from trauma. Search for 'Guide To Healing From Past Trauma'

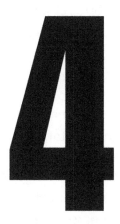

HOW TO
'CHILL OUT'
PROPERLY

Mind-Body Techniques
For Stress Reduction

Meditation practice isn't about trying to throw ourselves away and become something better. It's about befriending who we are already

— Pema Chödrön[10]

She sits crossed-legged on a patch of lush green grass seamed by willow trees, peacefully swaying in the light breeze. A breeze so gentle, it playfully sweeps thin strands of her long dark hair, loosely tied in a bun, across her face, tugging at her blouse and her palazzo pants, falling softly over her bare feet.

She is overlooking a pond, and while her eyes are closed, she is aware of the life the water sustains. Oh yes, this is evident by the cheerful chatter of birds nesting in the long reeds on the other side. Then there is also, every now and then, the plopping sound of a fish popping its head from below to hungrily grab mid-flight, a bug hovering above the surface.

It is an image of calmness and peace, radiating external serenity, but it also reflects the inner landscape she has established through meditation.

While this image is a beautiful reflection of what it means to meditate, it is often a wrongful impression many have of what meditation entails. It keeps too many from exploring this ancient practice as it appears so exclusive, a perception that often puts meditation out of reach for the average person. The image entices the mind with its serene nature. But a lack of understanding of meditation discourages many from even attempting this practice as it may appear impossible to achieve in a hurried lifestyle within the parameters of city living.

The latter is a myth this chapter will crush as meditation is a significantly effective way to utilize the mind-body connection to establish inner peace amidst external conflict and stress.

Meditation has many faces, and we'll explore how you can integrate the ancient practice into your modern lifestyle to restore internal harmony. But first, meditation's success is founded in the mind-body connection, a bond you need to understand to use it optimally to your benefit.

WHAT IS THE MIND-BODY CONNECTION?

The mind-body connection enables the mind to impact the body and the body to instigate change in the mind. It is a two-way street of possibility to initiate instant relief and establish long-term control over your body's stress response. The mind-body connection is so closely rooted in the nervous system that some may even perceive it as the nervous system.

It has been a point of discussion between philosophers for ages. But it is only recently that neuroscientists could determine the existence of this connection, how it functions, and how you can apply this connection to your gain.

Studying endless pages of academic documents capturing the results of many of these studies led me to understand how our thoughts and perspectives on life determine our physical state and health. It became evident that deliberately thinking positive thoughts and uplifting ideas can reduce internal stress levels while pondering on all the negative things in life increases the stress you experience.

Have you ever felt that even minor discomforts can become severely painful when your mind dwells on the negative? Or how a good bout of laughter can improve your physical symptoms, like relieving a headache? These things happen because this vital connection links mind and body into a complex network of fused systems.

We've learned from this research that emotions may manifest as thoughts in your mind, but due to the work of the nervous system, these thoughts manifest physically as feelings. Yes, indeed, the word *feeling* already indicates that thoughts have a physical impact, causing us to *feel* things even though they originated in the mind.

Today we know with absolute certainty that the mind can cause sensations and feelings in the body, and we can use the body to bring about change in the mind, too. Now, we're left to expand on these findings by exploring the practical techniques to optimize this feature[11].

MEDITATION VS. MINDFULNESS

Considering mindfulness and meditation as synonymous terms is a common misperception in the broader public. What makes it even easier to confuse is that you can increase mindfulness through meditation, and mindfulness is necessary to enter a meditative state. While the two terms are deeply infused, they remain separate entities. Furthermore, mindful meditation is another independent term contributing to the confusion.

But soon, the cloud of confusion will give way to an in-depth understanding of meditation, mindfulness, and how to practice both beneficially. Then you can use these tools to defend yourself against stress's impact on your life, relationships, happiness, and success. Once you've worked through each of these terms, exploring them in detail, you'll be equipped to alleviate the stress you feel at this very moment immediately.

We can loosely define meditation as a practice employing mind, body, brain, and behavior in a quiet location without distraction, where you can focus your attention to still the mind by focusing on a specific thought, thing, or element to establish an open attitude and a calm state of mind and body.

In comparison, a similar definition of mindfulness already reflects how meditation and mindfulness are similar but differ. Mindfulness refers to employing greater awareness of the sensations and experiences in the present moment to establish focus, increase joy and satisfaction, and establish a state of peace and calm in the mind and body.

You can employ mindfulness throughout the day, anywhere and anytime. Meditation is practiced for a specific set time daily. Mindfulness seeks greater awareness of every sensation, stimulation, object, vision, sound, and smell exposed to at the moment. Meditation shifts the focus beyond all these triggers to discipline the mind to focus on one thing alone. Mindfulness can be practiced during morning jogging, sitting at your desk, driving your car, or eating a meal. Meditation is best practiced in a quiet space where you can spend a set time undisturbed. There are many types of meditation to choose from when seeking the perfect practice to seek relief from your stress levels, but there is only one way to become more mindful.

Both mindfulness and meditation rely on using the body to quiet the mind for greater inner peace and calm. An added bonus is that you can benefit from all three mentioned practices through regular practice. You'll become empowered by turning them into a daily habit. No longer will you be on defense to make it through the day. No, you'll be empowered to face your days and the challenges they bring with courage and calmness. It equates to stepping into a desired position that appeared out of reach for far too long. I believe you're keen to step into your power and break free from the grip of stress.

MINDFUL MEDITATION

A discussion centering on meditation and mindfulness won't be complete without touching on what mindfulness meditation is too.

If you are new to meditation, mindfulness meditation offers a fantastic platform to get you started, requiring only a few simple and easy steps. The biggest challenge you may face is the demand for diligence and commitment to turn this practice into a habit. It is a disciplined practice combining elements of mindfulness and meditation to slow down your thoughts, lower your stress and anxiety levels, and restore a state of peace and calm in the body.

Like any other form of meditation, this type is a known method to switch off the SNS. Essentially, your breathing and deliberately taking control of the mind activates the PSNS to induce the physiological process to restore calm.

Yet, breathing isn't the only way to initiate change in the nervous system, causing it to transition from a state controlled by the SNS to where the PSNS is in charge. It is also possible by employing greater awareness.

Some benefits from mindfulness meditation include a slower heart rate and lowered blood pressure. Both these improvements benefit your cardiovascular system and reduce the risk of heart disease, strokes, or high blood pressure. We have researchers in alternative and complementary medicine to thank for a lot of what we know today about the benefits linked to mindfulness meditation. Over several years, if not decades, numerous studies have explored the impact of mindfulness-based stress reduction as a tool to improve stress management[12].

These studies demonstrated that mindfulness meditation reduces stress and mental health concerns accompanying high stress. I am specifically referring here to depression and anxiety. But did you know that persistently high-stress levels can lead to chronic pain? Participants of these studies noticed a significant improvement in the chronic pain they've been experiencing, making pain reduction an added benefit to mindfulness meditation.

Remember I mentioned that during the stress response controlled by the SNS, blood circulation is diverted away from several systems that aren't directly linked to offering protection from immediate threats, like the immune system? As a result, the immune system deteriorates due to a lack of nutrients and sufficient oxygen supply, causing it to become less effective, increasing the severity and shortening the intervals between bouts of illness. It means that mindfulness meditation is a tool to strengthen immune function, reducing the threat of illness.

Another benefit is that this state of greater calm improves sleep quality and eases the impact of insomnia on your holistic health.

So, the benefits are plenty; these are merely the highlights of what was determined through several studies. However, why not try it yourself? In your Workbook, you'll see space and relevant prompts to document your physical, mental, and emotional state to record your overall improvement.

Don't shy away from practicing mindful meditation. Rather, proceed to the practice as it is through practical application that you'll gain familiarity with the concept and enjoy its beneficial impact on your life. You can find a teacher or a program to follow, but practicing mindfulness meditation is easy. So, you can fly solo, get familiar with it, and become very good at it while practicing at your own pace.

One of the advantages of mindfulness meditation is you don't need to source any equipment before jumping in.

You don't need special candles (or any candles at all, for that matter), props, essential oils, or mantras. These things can make the experience more enjoyable but aren't requirements.

You need a quiet space to sit undisturbed for a few minutes; as little as 3-5 minutes are enough during the early stages. And you'll have to be open-minded, willing to be transformed to enjoy the life you desire. Lastly, a timer will be a helpful aid to keep you from watching the clock.

1. Choose an environment where you feel naturally at peace. This can be indoors or outside, but it should be quiet and disturbance-free for at least a few minutes.

2. Settle in a comfortable position. You can sit or lie down.

3. Set your timer for how long you want to practice, then forget about time.

4. Close your eyes and breathe deeply.

5. Set your intention for the session — to enter a state of internal calm.

6. Inhale deeply, taking note of the sensation as the air passes through the airways into your lungs. As you exhale, notice how your chest cavity contracts, squeezing out the air.

7. Thoughts may (most likely will) enter your mind. Acknowledge and let them go.

8. When your mind has wandered, bring it back and return your focus to breathing. Stay in the moment.

9. Once done, employ your heightened awareness to notice how different you feel mentally and physically.

Once you've practiced this stress-management technique and become skilled in using it to control your stress, it can be a vital aid to help you conquer your chronic stress levels.

BREATHING FOR STRESS RELIEF

"Just breathe" is often advice you would give someone visibly overwhelmed by external factors. It may even be that you use this line on yourself when feeling

overwhelmed, but have you ever pondered the physiological processes taking place when you do? Or, why breathing is such an effective antidote to stress?

What is essentially implied when instructed just to *breathe* is that you have to focus on slowing down your breathing, which can be done by taking deliberate deep breaths. This type of breathing is sometimes called *belly breathing*, as once you can feel your abdomen move up and down with every breath, you can be sure you're doing this effectively and can expect the promised results.

Breathing practices have been a trusted aid to improve a range of health concerns, like asthma, for ages. You may also be familiar with *pranayama* (praa-nuh-yaa-muh), a type of breathing used in yoga. Several methods of pranayama are applied in meditation and yoga. While yogis have relied on pranayama and its benefits for centuries, it is only as recent as the early 1800s when breathing exercises were introduced to the Western world[13].

When we explore the vagus nerve, in chapter nine, we will go into much more detail about the physiological processes taking place during periods of deep and deliberate breathing, but for now, let's seek instant gratification by adjusting your breathing style. It is a tool bringing instant relief to a stressed state, and you can also make this a daily habit to enjoy sustained results.

BREATHING TECHNIQUES

There are many ways to breathe to ensure relief, but I wanted to share the steps of a couple of methods to give you enough guidance to proceed independently.

THE PURSED LIP TECHNIQUE

The method forces you to slow down rapid and shallow breathing, typical of being trapped in the stress response.

1. Find a comfortable position to sit in.

2. Relax your shoulders and neck muscles.

3. While keeping your lips sealed, inhale for four counts through your nose.

4. Pucker your lips as if to blow out a candle and slowly exhale for four counts.

5. Repeat this exercise daily 4-5 times.

EQUAL BREATHING

The key to successful breathing is sufficient focus to ensure it happens gradually and deliberately. This specific technique, also known as *Sama Vritti*, meaning "equal mental fluctuation" in Sanskrit, dates back ages, and due to the high level of concentration the method requires, it restores balance in your breathing and mind.

1. Find a comfortable position in a quiet space.

2. Breathe in and out through your nose a couple of times.

3. Then, begin counting while you inhale, while holding your breath, and when exhaling. Be sure that every stage is equally long.

4. You can choose to pause between exhaling and the next inhale (it is natural to pause between breaths).

5. Continue this timed breathing for five minutes.

SITALI BREATHING

This is another method rooted in yoga that deliberately intends to still the thoughts and establish mental relaxation. It means "soothing" in Sanskrit.

1. Sit in a comfortable position.

2. Stick out your tongue and curl the edges together. Not everyone can do this. So, if you can't, then purse your lips.

3. Inhale through your mouth and exhale through your nose.

4. Keep this up for about five minutes.

The key to success with breathing exercises is to focus on your breathing. Notice how the airflow feels as it enters or exits your airways, fills your lungs, and expands your chest cavity. You can even place your hands on your abdomen to feel how the air pushes your belly out, putting more pressure on your hands.

These breathing exercises help get you meditative but aren't limited solely to meditation. You can practice breathing exercises at work, behind your desk, in the boardroom, on the subway, or at home. It is a tool available to you any time of the day or night, and it only requires a few minutes of your devotion to instantly release your stress as the physiological process of deep breathing triggers the PSNS into action. The more regularly you practice breathing exercises, the greater the likelihood that your predominant state will be one of greater calm.

PROGRESSIVE MUSCLE RELAXATION

You're no stranger to the pressure and discomfort, often even pain, caused by the build-up of muscle stress. As long as the muscles remain tight, it suppresses circulation, avoiding a sufficient supply of nutrients and oxygen, while toxic waste material gets trapped in the muscle tissue, causing inflammation. Not a desired state to be in.

Edmund Jacobson developed progressive muscle relaxation (PMR) in the 1920s. This American doctor found that tensing muscles and deliberately releasing this tension encourage greater overall relaxation. As an added benefit, he also found the practice improves mental stress by helping the mind relax[13].

The benefits of making PMR a regular practice are similar to what mindfulness meditation offers and more.

It is an easy practice requiring about 15-20 minutes daily.

1. Find a comfortable position. You can either sit upright or lie down on your back. It is more important to choose a position you can remain comfortable in for the time being than the exact position you choose.

2. Set your intention to relax the entire body. Taking about five slow deep breaths will help.

3. The technique works from one end of the body to the other. So, we will start at your toes and work our way up to the crown of your head.

4. Point your toes. Stretch them forward and upward, hold the position for a few counts, and then let go.

5. Proceed to your ankles, stretching them in all directions, holding position, and then letting the muscles relax.

6. Next up are your calves. Stretch these muscles and hold them tight for a few counts before letting go, allowing them to go soft in relaxation.

7. Gradually, you'll work your way upward through every muscle group.

8. Once you've squeezed your thighs and clenched your buttocks, release the muscles and let go.

9. Now, jump to your hands and fingers. Spread your fingers open wide, hold the tension, and relax.

10. The same goes for all your muscle groups in your forearms, then your biceps.

11. You can jump to your abdomen to address your torso when you reach the neck and shoulder area.

12. Contract the abdomen muscles, hold, and let go.

13. Move your way through the chest area, holding your breath and exhaling, allowing the muscles around the chest cavity to relax.

14. When you reach your neck and shoulders, pull your shoulders towards your ears, hold the position, and let go.

15. Even your facial muscles need to be stretched. Pull your mouth, lift your brows, and squint your eyes, every time holding the tension for a couple of counts before relaxing the muscle group.

16. Once you've worked your way to your crown, take a few deep breaths, mindful of how much more relaxed your body is and calmer you feel.

17. Get up, and take on the challenges of the rest of your day from a state of deep inner calmness.

Sure, the method may require a little more time than most breathing exercises, but it is a highly effective tool to prevent insomnia or set the intention for your day in the morning.

It is easy to neglect to focus on breathing, yet, life depends on it. Now you know that breathing isn't only sustaining life but also an effective tool to improve your quality of life. It is also at the core of mindfulness and meditation. In both ways, you can use the mind-body connection to take control of your stress levels. Practicing any of the mentioned methods will improve your overall well-being as you'll feel your stress level plummet. But the lasting benefit comes from regular practice, as this will support holistic healing and ensure you maintain a state of calmness and clarity even when facing adversity.

 Your Workbook shows these practices built into a week of healthy, mindful activities. Go there now to get your practice started.

Breathing is one type of movement you can utilize to engage in more effective stress management, but what if you could use every muscle in your body to gain the necessary control to trigger the PSNS? Exercise is another helpful aid to your disposal to enjoy calmness and clarity even when you find yourself trapped in a stressed reality. And don't believe the myth that you must build up a sweat to break the grip of stress. In the next chapter, we're cracking this myth wide open, for there are many forms of exercise, even for the least athletic of all, to manage stress through movement.

5

USING YOUR BODY AS A TOOL TO CREATE CALM

Exercise And Movement For Melting Away Stress

Deep breaths are like little love notes to your body.

– Unknown

"Cheating bastard!" Sarah tosses her phone in her locker before slamming the door. For a moment, she notices other ladies in the changing room at her gym staring at her as her lacking ability to control her emotions creates quite a stir, but what does she care? She is sure some are homewreckers, too, with tight-fitting pants and short tops. She could never understand what is the attraction to a married man. And the fool? His promises mean nothing...nothing at all!

She is furious as she storms out into the equipment area. Sarah doesn't realize that her intense stress levels since she saw her cheating husband and *that woman* are fueling her anger.

Her entire life is upside down. She kicked him out, but they'll have to sell the house. Her beautiful home and the garden...she worked so hard to get the garden the way she wanted it to look. At work, things aren't any easier. The McCormick deal will make or break her brand, and she isn't sure where it is heading. If the deal falls through, it will take her entire business into the gutter and find its position next to her marriage. The only difference is that she has to tell her team they no longer have jobs, and the idea of doing that makes her feel sick.

When Sarah has her boxing gloves on, her shoulder muscles are in a spasm, her headache just won't go, and her throat feels somewhat raw today. Quite frankly, she feels exhausted and unsure of what she is doing here. Perhaps she just wanted to punch something as she couldn't punch him, or maybe the gym appeared safer than going to an empty home filled with (now hollow) memories.

Sarah is unaware of the complexity of the system controlling the havoc in her body and mind. Or how her stress level increases her physical vulnerability. The stressful events in Sarah's life triggered the SNS, and she has been trapped in the stress response for quite some time. It is what is causing her fatigue, headache, and muscle spasms. Due to prolonged exposure to this high-stress state, her immune system is failing, hence the sore throat. Sarah came to the gym to escape her life, but over the next 30 minutes, she punched the living daylights out of the punching bag, and her body is taking giant leaps toward recovery.

WHY EXERCISE SHOULD BE IN YOUR STRESS MANAGEMENT TOOLBOX

Maybe you, too, want to punch something, believing it will ease your stress. Or perhaps, you have to walk from the boardroom table before losing your cool between colleagues. It can even be your kids and their constant bickering, driving you insane, and all you want to do is to pack your bags and run away as you can't take it anymore. Your home should be your safe haven, where you can rest and recuperate, but it might have just turned into a place keeping you trapped in stress and working long hours as you can hardly afford the ever-increasing mortgage.

Countless new stressful situations may bombard you daily, and this is overwhelming, to say the least. But the good news I share is that there is a solution to every stressful situation. There are many ways to ensure proper stress management, supporting holistic wellness. While exercise isn't the only way to employ the mind-body connection, it is an effective aid as it requires the power of full-body cooperation.

By learning more about the range of positive reactions you unleash by moving your body and what type of exercise works best, you can gain complete control over your life even while facing these stressful conditions.

NEURON GROWTH AND MAINTENANCE

Sarah works every muscle during her boxing session, giving her body a great combination of cardio and strength training. The cardio is increasing her heart rate, causing circulation to speed up. More blood is reaching her brain, providing extra oxygen and nutrients. This triggers her brain to release protein. This protein keeps her neurons healthy and supports her nervous system. But maintenance of the system controlling every aspect of your life is merely one of the benefits of getting active.

FEEL-GOOD HORMONES

But it isn't only her brain releasing helpful aids. No, the exercise also triggers her body to release a surge of dopamine and endorphins. You know these are the feel-good hormones, ensuring that when Sarah leaves the gym, she'll be floating on a cloud of positivity, a refreshing pause after spending most of the past couple of weeks wrapped in a haze of negativity. In contrast to the aggressive way she left in the locker room, she can now smile at a lady as they pass each other at the door.

EXCRETING TOXINS

She rapidly plants every punch, causing her body to heat up. Her body responds with excessive sweating to regulate her internal temperature. The activity instigates the release of toxins to be washed away by the bloodstream and excreted through her rapid breathing and sweating. Sarah may never know that the toxins she shed today would've caused inflammation in her muscles and impacted her overall wellness a couple of weeks from now had she not cleared her body from this poison.

AN EXERCISE "HIGH"

Cannabinoid (*ka-nuh-buh-noyd*) is the active ingredient in marijuana, causing the feeling of being high. A similar chemical, endocannabinoids (*en-doh-ka-nuh-buy-noydz*), can be found in the brain. The amygdala, which you are familiar with now, and the prefrontal cortex, another distinct area in the brain, are rich in endocannabinoid receptors.

For the longest time, researchers focused on how the increased release of dopamine and endorphins during exercise enhances mood. But now their focus has shifted to the release of endocannabinoids and how they reduce anxiety and instigate a state of contentment once locked into these receptors.[15].

Another benefit of this lasting high is that it improves how you respond to others. It becomes easier to connect with others, meaning that Sarah might have responded vastly differently after a session in the gym if she got the call from her soon-to-be ex now.

REGULAR EXERCISE MAKES YOUR BRAIN FIT FOR JOY

Exercise triggers your brain to be more hopeful, anticipate joy, and feel more motivated. When coupled with the increased levels of dopamine, regular exercise makes your brain fit for joy in the sense that your capacity to experience joy expands while depression levels plummet. This process serves well to combat the damage substance abuse can cause to brain chemicals. Drugs and other illegal substances alter brain chemicals and lower the natural dopamine level, but exercise can turn the tables on this state.

IMPROVES BRAIN BALANCE

The worst part of working yourself hard in the gym is the muscle pain in the next few days. This pain is caused by lactate, a byproduct of exercise, gathered in the muscle tissue. Recent research revealed that the negative light that illuminated lactate for so long is a rather unnecessary negative approach. Scientists found that lactate also makes a valuable contribution to brain health. Lactate travels to the brain, altering neurochemistry to alleviate anxiety and combat depression[15].

THE MOST EFFECTIVE TYPES OF EXERCISE TO LOWER YOUR STRESS LEVELS

Any form of exercise is better than no exercise, but if your goal is to use your fitness routine to combat your stress levels, some forms stand out. What makes these better than others? It is hard to pinpoint a specific feature setting a form of exercise apart, as success largely depends on finding the perfect combination of breathing and intensity for your body and unique needs. If we have to look at an umbrella term to direct you towards success, I would say seek exercise categorized as moderate to intense. But that said, we have yoga at the top of the list, highlighting the importance of effective breathing while increasing activity!

YOGA

Yoga is a fantastic form of exercise to reduce stress and anxiety. The stress-reducing power of yoga is locked in the combination of controlled breathing and posture exercises. The duo of features encourages relaxation and recovery as it activates the PSNS. So, sure, you can choose more intense forms of exercising (don't underestimate yoga's intensity), but if you're not athletic, don't shy away from all forms of exercise. You can boost your brain and bring inner calm without getting into your jogging shoes.

RESISTANCE TRAINING

Resistance training is an excellent boost for your confidence as you'll gradually be able to pick up heavier weights, increasing your trust in your abilities to overcome all kinds of obstacles. Studies also indicate that if you keep up a regular resistance training routine twice a week, you'll notice a considerable improvement in anxiety symptoms and far fewer worries consuming your mind[15]. You don't have to hit the gym for resistance training, so don't let the idea of sweating in public put you off training. Squats, push-ups, and sit-ups at home will suffice.

AEROBIC EXERCISES

Under aerobic exercises, we can include any activity that will have you gasping for air. Swimming, dancing, jogging, roller-skating, and spinning are some options. This exercise boosts the release of endorphins to leave you feeling great. Most exercises in this category also bring unique individual benefits, like swimming and dancing.

- Swimming requires complete submersion, which is therapeutic, while repeating the strokes helps increase focus.

- Dancing is lovely for getting your heart pumping on several levels. The activity will speed up your heart rate, but being close to a dancing partner causes the release of oxytocin (*ok-suh-tow-sn*) to spike. While this is the hormone that stimulates contractions during labor, an increased level of the hormone reduces blood pressure and cortisol levels.

BRISK WALKING IN GREEN SPACES   *So good!*

Brisk walking is an aerobic exercise, but I want to distinguish this form of exercise as it is happening in a green space. Spending time in green spaces is gradually becoming a better-known form of stress reduction to ensure mental health.

Green spaces refer to any outdoor environment where you are surrounded by nature. Spending time in these spaces can lower your stress levels, improve cognitive functioning, and increase your attention span. Nature remains the go-to destination to enhance your overall mental well-being most effectively. It provides an escape from the rushed lifestyle and the perfect setting for reflection or introspection. In chapter nine, I expand more on *forest bathing*, an excellent way to reap the most benefits green spaces offer.

ENGAGE IN TEAM SPORTS

Team sports have to be on the list as there are also multiple benefits you can enjoy from engaging in this type of activity. Sure, you'll enjoy the same release of feel-good hormones, but strengthening your bonds with your teammates or competitors is an added benefit. Team sports provide a sense of belonging, which also contributes to improved stress management.

MINDFUL MOVEMENT PRACTICES

So, I've already touched on yoga, being at the top of the list of effective ways to engage your body through the mind-body connection to improve your mental state. That said, there are several other options to consider, falling in the mindful movement category.

It may come as a surprise, as it is so commonly assumed that mindful movement is limited to practices like yoga or tai chi, but any form of exercise can constitute a mindful movement. When it comes to this type of workout, it isn't as much about what you do but how you do it.

Whether you ride a bike, lift weights in the gym, or ski down snow-covered slopes, these activities can all count as mindful movement. How? When deliberately breathing in a manner that encourages the mind to transition from being stressed and distracted to feeling strong and capable. Regardless of what type of activity you prefer to get your blood pumping, as long as you do it mindfully and remain aware in the present moment, it would count as mindful movement. The key to success is ensuring that whenever your mind wanders to stressful situations or occasions, you acknowledge that it happened and bring it back to the present moment and what you're doing.

As mindful movement is such a vast range of activities, it is probably best explained by dividing it into four categories.

BREATHING EXERCISES

The breathing exercises I refer to differ from the typical slow deep breaths you would take during mindful meditation. This exercise group refers to purposefully using your breath to address mental health concerns through the mind-body connection. It means taking, at times, slow and deep breaths to activate the PSNS and, at times, switching to short rapid breathing if you want to sharpen your focus and refresh your mind.

WALKING MEDITATION

Don't confuse walking meditation with brisk walking in nature. When you go for a walk, whether a stroll or at a faster pace, the intention is to get your heart rate up and blood pumping. It is considered a form of physical exercise in which a targeted time or distance is usually linked. During walking meditation, you use the mind-body connection to establish a state of inner calm and focus through movement and awareness. There is no estimated timeframe or distance to cover. The intention isn't to walk fast but rather to walk deliberately. Deliberately? What does that mean? While walking, focus on your breathing, notice the feeling of the ground underneath your feet, and be aware of every muscle that is contracting, stretching, or relaxing as you step forward. When you realize your mind is wandering, slowly bring it back to enjoy greater awareness.

STRETCHING EXERCISES

Yoga is a stretching exercise, but stretching isn't limited to yoga. You can use many other stretches to release stress and negative emotions trapped in the body. The reality of many people's lives today is that long hours are spent sitting in front of a computer. When the body isn't moving enough, it becomes stiff, and this discomfort removes your focus and concentration. Simply getting up from behind the screen, and stretching your arms, back, shoulders, and legs right where you are, is a way to use your body and movement to refresh your mind and increase your energy. You will feel revitalized and will be able to persevere much longer.

OTHER FORMS OF EXERCISE

Every type of physical activity or exercise you can think of can be turned into a mindful movement when you utilize training to synchronize your breathing while being aware of the processes in your body.

Whether you're thirsty and go to the kitchen for a glass of water or need to relieve yourself from that water a short while later and get up to go to the bathroom, your body's needs are handled effectively by taking action. Why would it be any different for the mind? When it comes to mental stress, anxiety, and even depression, and you need to uplift your mind and soul, you can achieve the desired relief by taking action too.

In this case, action would constitute the exercise required to sustain your mental health. We've discovered several great forms of movement that can bring about many benefits, but one more type of movement hasn't been addressed—the movement of our jaws. Meet me in the next chapter to explore eating. Discover the impact of how, when, and what you eat on healthy stress management.

 But first, spend some time with your Workbook, where you'll see precisely how and when you can squeeze in all these health-boosting, stress-management exercises.

6

FOOD TO FUEL YOUR FLOW

The Role Of Nutrition In Stress Reduction

The road to health is paved with good intestines.

– Sherry A. Rogers[16]

He loads as much as possible onto his fork with a nifty hand movement. Perfectly directed for his mouth, the fork is cleared with one big bite. Bravo! It is all in. It crunches as he chews while his gaze remains fixated on the screen before him. Several seconds passed before a droplet of sauce on his hand resting next to the bowl on his desk brought his attention to the fact that the last bite didn't go as smoothly as he thought. He grabs a napkin to wipe his chin, and his focus returns to the words on the screen.

Jason is one of the millions of people with daily lunch breaks at their desks. The modern-day pressure often doesn't allow for lengthy lunches followed by a brisk walk back to the office. However, Jason is slightly different. His fork is loaded with a crispy salad, and the sauce on his chin is low-fat salad dressing. A recent firm warning from his doctor convinced Jason to address his obesity. Now, he is *committed* to healthy eating, sticking to low-calorie foods.

While the meal fills him, a mere few minutes later, he walks past the staff kitchen and notices a display of freshly baked pastries. Instantly, his mouth is watering, and he can feel his stomach growl. But he just ate; how is this even possible?

There is a saying that *the way to a man's heart is through his stomach*. I don't know if that's always true, but I know the mind-body connection is the highway between the gut and the brain, and how well you control the traffic impacts your stress management.

UNDERSTANDING THE GUT-BRAIN AXIS

To understand how the gut impacts the brain, we should start by exploring how the brain affects the gut. The latter is, after all, an effect impacting our lives daily. I am referring to the sensation of hunger. So, let's dig into digestion and how hunger is triggered in the brain rather than being a gut sensation.

The precise timing depends on what you had during your last meal, but it takes about 2 - 5 hours until all the food in your stomach is digested[17]. While food will still be in the digestive tract for quite some time, the content in the stomach has cleared out. This movement is controlled by contractions known as the migrating movement complex (MMC). A hormone, motilin, controls the final stages of clearing the stomach. Motilin also triggers hunger pangs, indicating the body is ready to consume more food. Yet, motilin isn't the only hormonal roleplayer causing the need to eat.

Ghrelin activates neurons in the hypothalamus, telling you you're hungry. Your ghrelin level peaks when you're hungry and is the highest before eating. Eating causes this level to drop, resulting in a fading sensation of hunger. It will usually stay low for about an hour after eating, but once your stomach becomes empty, the level gradually increases, indicating an increasing need for food[18].

Yet, Jason immediately needed to eat again when he saw the pastries. What happened there?

Essentially, the body communicates hunger through the brain-gut axis in two ways. So, there are two types of hunger. A *homeostatic hunger* is one you satisfy during regular meals, indicating that the body needs to replenish its energy resources. *Hedonic hunger* is considered an opportunistic attempt of the body to cash in on additional energy supplies once noticed—like freshly baked pastries, low in nutrients, easily digested, and energy-dense, smelling amazingly mouthwatering.

Our knowledge about hedonic hunger is much more limited as it isn't nearly as well-researched as homeostatic hunger. But we know the following things:

- You'll resist hedonic hunger and walk away from temptation if you are able to maintain a low-calorie intake.

- If your brain is committed (hard-wired) to seek additional energy constantly, you're far more likely to grab a bite.

- If your last meal satisfies you, the temptation triggered by hedonic hunger will be short-lived, and it can be an easy pass.

Now, we can wonder what Jason did, but let's rather proceed to explore the brain-gut axis, for if the brain can impact the gut in this profound way, the gut has the same effect on the brain too. The latter is a topic that researchers only more recently began to explore to determine the impact of gut health on mental, physical, and emotional wellness[19]. When grasping the state of gut health's powerful influence on the brain, statements like *going with your gut, butterflies in the stomach,* and calling the gut *the second brain* make much more sense.

The gut has its own nervous system, called the enteric (*in-the-rukh*) nervous system (ENS). Does the name ring a bell? I've mentioned it in chapter two, as it is part of the larger autonomic nervous systems with the SNS and PSNS.

The ENS consists of two thin layers in the gastrointestinal (digestive) tract, tallying more than 100 million nerve cells. It is spread across the entire area, from the esophagus to the rectum. The ENS isn't capable of having independent thought, but it is in constant communication with the CNS (central nervous system). This line of communication is the axis between the gut and the brain. It is how digestive concerns like irritable bowel syndrome can cause emotional changes, a phenomenon so influential, research indicates people with bowel problems are significantly more prone to depression and anxiety[20].

But this isn't the end of the gut's impact on your mood yet. It also controls 95% of the body's serotonin production[20]. Without a healthy gut, your entire body's homeostasis can be disturbed, leaving you feeling sick but, even more importantly, stressed and miserable.

The gut's duties include

- digestion and metabolism regulation

- vitamin and nutrient uptake from food

- programming the immune system

- keeping outside invaders at bay by building and maintaining the gut wall

- blocking harmful microbes and keeping them from invading your system

- producing antimicrobial chemicals protecting the body against pathogens

If gut health deteriorates and slips up on just one of the above responsibilities, your entire system, including your mental health, will be impacted.

Until now, most research has been conducted on mice and other animals to explore how much gut health contributes to mental health. Still, the findings are so profound it encourages many more studies to map the exact nature of the brain-gut axis. That said, we can say with absolute certainty that gut health contributes to a stressed mind and that we can and should optimize this link to use nutrition to establish more effective stress management.

NUTRITION AND STRESS MANAGEMENT: WHAT YOU SHOULD KNOW

Nutrition should always be understood as the necessity to provide the body with what it needs to grow and remain healthy. Remember, this isn't the same as eating. Eating includes all types of food, but not all foods are sources of nutrition. A large part of the typical modern-day diet includes food sources high in calories but low in nutrition. It is helpful to be selective in what you include in your diet, as this will impact gut health, causing a ripple effect on your mental and emotional states.

When looking at food with a more discerning eye, it becomes clear what food you should include to supply your body's demand for nutrition. This insight will guide you to what to eat to sustain gut health and better manage stress via the brain-gut axis.

The number of different eating styles and diet options being promoted can be overwhelming. But one way of eating stands out above all others, considering stress management — the Mediterranean diet. Why? Because it includes a balanced selection of food containing anti-inflammatory properties. By reducing inflammation, you lower cortisol levels and, as a direct result, stress levels. But there is more to it.

When we dissect the Mediterranean diet to explore what it includes and why it is so effective, it is evident that the food types part of this way of eating brings abundant benefits to your overall well-being and supports effective stress management. See for yourself.

B VITAMINS

All B vitamins have a crucial role, but vitamin B12 is essential in breaking down cortisol. B vitamins also produce and regulate dopamine and serotonin neurotransmitters, ensuring good-mood management.

Food sources high in B vitamins are often derived from animal protein. Still, there are plenty of options for vegetarians and vegans too:

- Eggs
- Chicken
- Beef
- Fish

- Milk and dairy products
- Nutritional yeast
- Fortified breakfast cereals

OMEGA-3 FATTY ACID

When a 2011 research study found a positive correlation between the consumption of foods high in omega-3 fatty acids and a mentionable reduction in anxiety, it opened the doors to much greater interest and research exploring the benefits of including the nutrient in your diet to aid in stress management[21].

Omega-3 fatty acids reduce inflammation and so contribute to better stress management. Yet, this nutrient's most influential contribution is its ability to cross the blood-brain barrier. What this means is that it can impact brain cells directly. Omega-3 is valuable in sustaining growth, maintenance, and supporting cell renewal. Direct cell support combats the impact of stress on nerve cells and so effectively supports stress management[22].

Foods containing high levels of omega-3 fatty acids are:

- Oily fish like anchovies, mackerel, sardines, herring, salmon, and tuna
- Seeds, specifically chia and sesame
- Olive oil

- Avocado

- Walnuts

MAGNESIUM

Due to magnesium's role in breaking down cortisol and reducing inflammation, it is an essential building block in any stress management plan.

Foods to consider adding to your diet are:

- Banana
- Avocado
- Spinach

- Pumpkin seeds
- Broccoli
- Dark chocolate

PROTEIN

Protein has many more roles in health management than merely being a fundamental building block in muscle tissue.

A high adrenaline level linked to being stressed triggers the release of sugar into circulation to ensure the body has sufficient energy to protect itself. It is a helpful aid if the threat is real but a dangerous state to remain in for extended periods, like when experiencing acute stress. Persistent high blood sugar holds the potential to trigger a range of secondary but severe health concerns. It is where protein is helpful as an increased protein uptake stabilizes blood sugar and combat the impact of stress on overall health and wellness.

Protein-rich food sources are high in tryptophan (*trip-tuh-fan*). The body itself can't produce tryptophan, an amino acid needed to produce serotonin. Serotonin is a feel-good hormone, and its role is evident in stress management. Serotonin is also required to produce melatonin. When the body is exposed to low-light conditions, like at night, serotonin is triggered to make melatonin, sustaining the sleep/wake cycle and combating insomnia[23]. So, including enough protein in your diet is vital to support a good mood and healthy sleeping patterns.

While the conventional perception of protein-rich food sources is often limited to animal protein, plenty of alternative plant-based options exist. When choosing animal protein, it is important to include lean meats to prevent the intake of empty calories contained in the fat.

- Chicken breast
- Lean beef
- Eggs
- Turkey breast
- Salmon
- Shrimp

- Tuna
- Lentils
- Beans
- Almonds
- Quinoa
- Peanuts

FERMENTED FOODS

Gut health depends on a balanced intake of fermented foods, sustaining the good microbes to allow the gut to function optimally. These are foods high in probiotics, creating a healthy environment for the gut to function optimally.

The palette of the masses may not prefer fermented foods, but you don't need to consume them in high volumes to reap the benefits they bring, supporting the brain-gut axis.

- Kimchi
- Sauerkraut
- Greek yogurt
- Kefir
- Tempe
- Miso
- Natto

Wait! I forgot to add Kombucha!

FOODS TO AVOID

Including these foods in your diet will sustain the gut health necessary to support the brain-gut axis in effective stress management. But just like these foods are vital to include in your diet, certain foods severely impact the gut, combatting all the good these foods contribute to support gut health.

Foods you need to limit and preferably avoid completely are:

- alcohol

- soda

- high-sugar foods

- simple carbs like pasta, cake, and white flour

As important as what you eat is when you eat, how often you eat, and how much you eat is mindful eating.

MINDFUL EATING PRACTICES

Mindful eating improves digestion and supports gut health to remain an effective roleplayer combatting stress. So, if eating nutritional food is the main act in the play, helping the brain-gut axis to manage stress, then mindful eating is the supporting act. It is a process requiring awareness while you eat, to be present in the moment, experiencing every bite through all the senses. The way Jason was having lunch at the start of the chapter is in direct contrast to mindful eating. While he did try to lower his calorie intake, he failed to the extent that his play lacked this vital supporting act.

Through mindful eating, you improve your awareness of healthy eating. Following a nutritional diet and managing cravings become easier. It is a way to actively shift your attention to a non-judgmental approach toward nutrition to support the mind-body connection. The result is limited digestive problems and a reduction in problematic eating habits.

Mindful eating triggers the PSNS, improving several causes of digestive concerns. It increases circulation to the digestive system, enhances nutrient absorption, improves peristalsis and MMC, and limits nausea, stomach aches, vomiting, and diarrhea. These benefits include increased enzymes, gastric juice, bile release, and ensuring optimal digestion while enjoying resting and inner calm[24].

TIPS TO PRACTICE MINDFUL EATING

Mindful eating starts during the preparation and plating of your food. Make it appealing, add color and variety to the plate, and present it mouthwateringly.

- When sitting down, take time to smell the flavors and aromas of the food.

- Notice your hunger, how it affects your body, and how having this plate in front of you affects your body physically.

- Every bite is a taste sensation, so notice the different textures and tastes on your fork.

- Take a moment to consider the origin of your food, who prepared it, and how it was prepared while being grateful for being able to enjoy the meal.

- Eat slowly and remain aware of how the food makes you feel. Notice when you're feeling satisfied and have had enough.

- Consider the nutrients in your meal and how this helps to maintain your body, supporting your health.

- Reflect on why you chose this meal, how it impacts you, and the effect having this meal has on the environment.

We live in a world thirsting for instant gratification. Modern society tends to jump to easy solutions and quick fixes to resolve every challenge. It is why many people opt for pharmaceuticals to address their challenges when their stress levels are out of control. Yet, the solutions to many of life's challenges are already inside us.

Have you ever considered something as simple as eating vital in effective stress management? Would you still need to reach out to chemicals to gain control over your life if you can do this simply by changing your eating habits? **!!!**

 To help you use the information above straight away in a tasty way, we've included a grocery shopping list and 19 recipes in your Workbook. Go there now to see what's on the menu!

Managing stress by taking care of the nervous system is a continuous process. Every choice you make will have a positive or negative outcome in this regard, whether you're eating or sleeping, as you'll see in the next chapter. Join me there to learn how your sleeping habits can contribute to effective stress management.

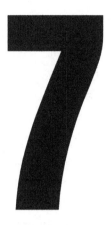

7

SNOOZE
YOUR WAY
TO PEACE

Why Sleep Is The Ultimate Path
To A Calmer Life

Happiness is a nice long nap.

– Peanuts[25]

Tick, tick, tick...how much noise can one tiny bit of plastic make? Every tick echoes in Craig's head. Every tick sounds like an explosion bouncing around inside his skull. Why does his wife, Jennifer, have to be so old school regarding alarm clocks? He wishes he knew. He has pondered it every night for the past couple of months. Since his company started restructuring, he has had very little sleep.

Initially, his concerns about his position becoming collateral damage in an attempt to save the business kept him awake night after night. Then, it was evident that his future at the firm had a gloomy outlook. Gradually, he could feel the tension in every fiber of his being. The situation took a dramatic nosedive when he lost his cool and punched his colleague, Bob. The situation escalated. Threats were flying. Craig was out of control. Security tased him when he picked up a cup to use to wipe the smirk off the schmuck's face. This is, of course, an update he hasn't shared with Jennifer yet. He is sure once he shares the news with her, he'll be all alone ... in this bed ... lying in silence ... staring at the ceiling ... without her soft breathing soothing him into eventual sleep ... even if just for an hour or two.

WHEN YOU DON'T SLEEP

The longest anyone has ever gone without sleep is 264 hours, equalling 11 days. Did the person die? No, there is no certainty about how long you can go without sleep before death steps in.[26] The body would go into a severe state of distress before that happens. Testing the limits of your own ability to go without sleep is never recommended.

We do know that after only 24 sleepless hours, the body will respond similarly to having a blood alcohol level of 0.10 %, which is well above the legal limit when driving. We also know that a lack of sleep lasting this long can alter your perceptions, reduce memory, cause tremors and irritability, and increase muscle tension.[26]

Many of the changes you experience mentally, physically, and emotionally result from the increase in the stress hormones, adrenaline, and cortisol that the body releases to help you cope with the lack of sleep.[27] Without rejuvenation through proper rest, the body takes an alternative approach to maintain functionality. As these hormones keep your body trapped in the stress response state, it is no surprise that after 36 hours of no sleep, there is a drastic increase in inflammatory markers in your bloodstream, contributing to high blood pressure and heart disease. It is typical for blood pressure to lower by roughly 10-20% while sleeping, a drop that doesn't occur while remaining in a sleepless state.[27]

Evidently, a lack of sleep can be disastrous on many levels, which poses the question of what happens to the nervous system while sleeping. And the spin-off from this enquiry is what you can do if sleep escapes you night after night.

SLEEP AND HOW IT SUPPORTS THE NERVOUS SYSTEM

Even today, the entire range of processes occurring in the mind and body while you're sleeping remains somewhat unclear. Yet, there are a lot of things we do know. This knowledge confirms that proper sleep is essential for adequate stress management.

SLEEP ALLOWS TIME TO PROCESS INFORMATION

Your mind is exposed to an immense amount of information throughout the day. As this is a continuous flow taking place for as long as you're awake, once you sleep and this exposure stops, your brain can actively start to process this information and store long-term memories. These would include the memories of notable events in your life, but it is also the basis of learning new skills and forming the foundation on which you build new knowledge.

HORMONAL MANAGEMENT

Your body releases several hormones while sleeping, including melatonin, which is vital to induce a sleepy state and make you feel drowsy.

These are all important processes during sleep, but the following three processes are of even greater importance in the quest for stress management.

THE SNS (SYMPATHETIC NERVOUS SYSTEM) GOES INTO A RESTING STATE

Sleep helps to shut down the stress response. So, even if you're constantly operating under the stress response when you awake, this stress response lets go of its grip and gives your body a break it needs. Therefore, if you don't get enough sleep, you're robbing your body of this opportunity to relax and putting it automatically in a state similar to the stress response, worsening the problem even further.

DECREASE IN STRESS HORMONES

While you're sleeping, cortisol levels drop naturally. As the cortisol level is intertwined in the stress response, triggering and maintaining this state of high alert, it is vital to give your body a break from this stress. Even if you wake up still trapped in the stress response, your body at least has to deal with lower cortisol levels while sleeping.

YOUR MUSCLES RELAX

Non-rapid eye movement sleep (NREM) and rapid eye movement sleep (REM) are the two predominant stages in the sleep cycle. During both stages, your muscles are completely relaxed and almost paralyzed to keep you from acting on your dreams and hurting yourself and others. This state of muscle relaxation ensures better blood circulation to your muscles, providing nutrients and oxygen while releasing toxins to be flushed out of your system. When the ideal environment never exists for these processes, muscle aches and pains will only worsen due to increased inflammation.

Quality sleep is an undeniable part of effective stress management. That brings us to the point where it is necessary to consider the quality of *your* sleep. Are you sleeping enough? Is it quality sleep you're getting? Is the sleep you get every night sufficient to cater for your needs?

The best way to determine whether you're enjoying quality sleep is by determining whether the five aspects of quality sleep are present in your sleeping habits. The acronym, SATED, summarizes these aspects.[28]

- **S**atisfaction refers to how satisfied you are with the sleep you get.

- **A**lertness demands that you rate how alert and refreshed you feel during the day.

- **T**iming questions whether there is consistency in the times you go to bed and wake up.

- **E**fficiency refers to how much of the time you're in bed you sleep.

- **D**uration determines whether you've gotten enough sleep.

All five of these characteristics must be present in your sleeping habits. If we revert to Craig's example, we can assume that his timing score will be adequate, he may even spend several hours in bed. But his satisfaction, alertness, duration, and efficiency are all lacking. Meeting one or two requirements is just not sufficient. Take a moment now to complete the SATED exercise in the Workbook to determine your sleep state.

A poor SATED score can increase stress, but it is also a result of poor stress management. The relationship between sleep and stress management can complement each other or be a vicious cycle spinning out of control. I can't overemphasize the need to address this concern if you're experiencing the latter. You can establish immense improvement in this regard by adopting healthy sleeping practices.

OPTIMAL SLEEP HYGIENE

Sleep hygiene is an umbrella term for an optimal environment and conditions to enjoy peaceful and uninterrupted sleep. It considers your bedroom, temperature, linen, schedule, and bedtime routine.

Five pillars support sleep hygiene.

- Value your sleep as an essential part of holistic health support.

- Prioritize sleep as part of stress management.

- Personalize your sleeping routine to support your unique requirements.

- Trust that once you've identified the perfect sleep window for your needs, it will bring the benefits you hope for.

- Protect your sleeping pattern. Set the necessary boundaries to ensure you can go to bed when needed.

Indications of poor sleep hygiene are when you're struggling to fall asleep, wake up often at night, or need to nap during the day. While other factors can also cause these concerns, it will be good practice to ensure your sleep hygiene is optimal before addressing other concerns.

STEPS TO OPTIMAL SLEEP HYGIENE

You can improve your sleep hygiene and support quality sleep by taking simple steps.

- Define your sleep schedule by going to bed and waking up at roughly the same time every day.

- Treat sleep like the priority it should be in your life. By this I mean avoid giving preference to having fun, screen time or working over sleeping.

- Daytime naps can be fun and are a real treat, but sleeping during the day can affect your sleep at night and be the reason you're struggling to fall asleep. So, if you struggle to fall asleep, cut back on your daytime naps.

- When making changes to your sleep routine, do it gradually. Creating any sudden transitions in this regard can overthrow your entire sleeping routine.

- A nighttime routine indicates to your brain what is about to happen to help it prepare for sleep by slowing down. It also helps to go to bed every night at the same time.

- Step away from electronic devices for at least 30 minutes (preferably longer) before you want to sleep. The blue light of these devices keeps your brain active and will prevent sleep. Instead, grab a book and read to relax your mind. _!!!_

- A warm shower or bath before bedtime can also help calm the mind and body.

- The environment (referring to your room and bed) should be comfortable and not too hot or cold. Some people prefer to sleep under heavy blankets, while others are quickly hot or feel suffocated by the weight on top of them. Choose bed linen, like natural linen, that can absorb sweat and regulate your temperature to support uninterrupted sleep.

- Refrain from making any mental connections linked to activity with your bedroom. It means that it is best to keep your bedroom for what it is intended, sleeping or as a place to relax. If you're in the habit of bringing work to bed, you're establishing a mental connection that your bedroom is a place of work instead of rest. Take it a step further and keep your phone out of the bedroom too. Or, at least, out of the bed.

- Bright light can also keep sleep at bay, so opt for dim light to create a relaxing environment.

- Some precautions you can take to support good sleep start during the day. Ensure enough exposure to sunlight, as this helps your circadian (sur-key-dee-uhn) rhythm. Circadian rhythm refers to the mental, physical, and behavioral changes occurring in the body within a 24-hour cycle. These changes are regulated by exposure to light and darkness.

- An increased activity level also contributes to nighttime exhaustion and will help you to sleep better.

- Reducing or eliminating smoking, a known cause of poor quality sleep, will be helpful.

- Late-night dining requires digestion when the body should be allocating resources to functions other than digestion.

✗
- Alcohol may make you sleepy, but consuming alcoholic drinks close to bedtime will result in poor-quality sleep, keeping the body from entering a healthy sleeping cycle.

Once you have all of these in place, you can advance healthy sleeping practices by including mindful sleep practices in your routine.

MINDFUL SLEEPING PRACTICES

As mindful eating inevitably plays an essential role in effective stress management, so do mindful sleeping practices. Highly effective mindful sleeping practices include meditation, deep breathing exercises, meditative movement, and progressive relaxation. In chapter four, we've already gone into extensive detail about these practices, and I only want to emphasize the benefit of following these practices before bedtime. They'll contribute to quality sleep by encouraging deep relaxation on all levels.

A mindful sleeping practice still open for exploration is meditative movement.

MEDITATIVE MOVEMENT

Tai chi, yoga, and qigong (*chee-gong*) are all forms of this practice to instill a deep sense of calm and relaxation.

Of these practices, tai chi and qigong stand out as highly beneficial. Both are ancient techniques requiring no special equipment. They can be practiced at home. Tai chi can directly be translated as *meditation in motion*. Qigong and tai chi consist of gentle, slow, and controlled movements coupled with controlled breathing. These exercises improve flexibility, muscle strength, and coordination but also establish a state of emotional and mental calmness.

Meditative movements are easy to practice and require a small investment before bedtime to calm the mind and body, supporting quality sleep. I recommend you initially join a group or team up with an expert or instructor of any of these practices. Once you're comfortable doing it alone, nothing stops you from employing these forms of meditative movement as much as you like.

Missing out on relaxing and rejuvenating sleep has an immensely negative impact on your health and wellness, diminishing your chances of effective stress management. But you can vastly improve your sleep quality by making a few small changes in your sleeping habits and environment. It is how you can use sleep to manage your stress levels and take control of your nervous system's stress response.

So far, we considered the changes you can make when you shift your perspective. We've covered practices using the mind-body connection to improve stress management, exercise, and nutrition. Now, we explored the changes you can make to your sleeping routine to gain control over your stress management.

But what happens when you shift your focus away from the self and to your microenvironment, the people you spend time with, those who surround you, care for you and contribute to your life? You can even extend your glance to your meso and macro environments. Meso would be the top management of the company you work for, suppliers who are mere acquaintances or even your wider community you belong to. The people in your macro environment are lawmakers of your city, or country. I'll meet you in the next chapter for a closer review of your social support network, identifying who they are, how they contribute to your life, and how you can make the most of these connections.

 Before you move on, spend a moment in your Workbook to complete the exercises you'll find in there. They are highly relevant to this chapter and topic.

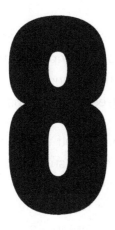

8

STRESS AND
THE FRIEND-FACTOR

**Your Social Circles Can Create
Or Damage Your World**

*If you want to go fast, go alone.
If you want to go far, go together.*

– African Proverb[29]

Do you speed through life and its moments, the pleasant ones and those less so, just to see what is next? Perhaps you're in a race to make more money, gain more popularity, or attend another social event. For you, life is a race from one hair-raising corner to the next. If this lifestyle suits you, you might like being a lone wolf. You move faster alone without the need to consider others while navigating through life, hurrying along at your own pace.

Yet, what you may find is that your life is unsatisfying. It may feel as though it always demands more of you to make it feel more rewarding. You have to keep pushing the boundaries until you're so consumed with chasing satisfaction, joy, and contentment that burnout becomes inevitable in your future. While you're running at full speed, you're missing the beauty along the way.

When you slow down a little, you'll experience quite a contrasting reflection of life. Then you'll see that life has so much more to offer. It isn't a race but a journey, a road trip designed to offer you a kaleidoscope of experiences, enriching your existence.

Road trips are always better when shared. Moving slower and with awareness of your surroundings allows you to belong to something much larger than yourself—you become part of a community and an environment. It becomes a far richer adventure feeding your soul, mind, and body.

These slow trips are the ones you take on with a travel companion. Travel companions ease the burden of hardships along the way. Companions make the stretches through barren landscapes feel shorter. At the same time, sharing your journey with others multiplies the magnificence of your experience. These companions are the ones who empower you to the very end of your trip.

Casey's story reveals how a greater awareness of your surroundings and the people who form part of it can guide you through challenges and how being connected to others can provide you with the support you need.

CASEY'S SOCIAL SUPPORT

"It is my anniversary," Casey protested.

"This company's success isn't founded on sweet little gatherings. Decide whether you want to be one of the best in your field or please your hubby with a home-cooked meal. You can't have both." Liz, the fashion house owner where Casey is carving out her career as a successful designer, is cold as ice. She has never married and doesn't have any family. Understanding this about Liz should indicate to Casey what to expect of the woman controlling her future in this firm.

"What do I do? I don't want to choose. Of course, I am serious about my career, but how do I tell Harry I can't make it to our dinner? He made the reservation months ago?" Casey is stressed, depressed, and only a few breaths away from bursting into tears. Her outburst occurs at her desk on the shoulder of her dear friend and office confidant, Sheila.

"Don't worry. Harry has got your back. I've seen how he treats you. He loves you, Casey, and he wouldn't want you to be so stressed about your celebration. Liz is an ice queen, but don't let her ruin your day. And by the way, congrats on the anniversary," Sheila says as she walks to her desk.

'Sheila is right. She always makes me feel better,' Casey thinks as she picks up the phone to call her husband.

Of course, Sheila makes Casey feel better. She is part of Casey's social support system, and thanks to research, we now know that this type of connection plays a crucial role in effective stress management.

During a 2022 study, the assumption that social support increases resilience and can help you overcome stressful situations with much greater ease was proven. For ages, people from all generations have enjoyed the benefits of friendships, of being kind to one another, but now we have research confirming what was suspected all along. Now we know for sure that loneliness is a contributing factor to declining mental health concerns, affecting your physical wellness too.[30]

THE CONNECTION BETWEEN SOCIAL SUPPORT AND STRESS MANAGEMENT

During tough times, few things offer as much comfort and relief as conversing with someone you care about and trust. These bonds provide a place to unburden your mind and de-stress yourself.

Social support offers benefits like reinforcing healthy habits. That said, it is only valid if you surround yourself with people disciplined in their own healthy habits. Either way, remember that your actions are mostly influenced by those who surround you. The more time you spend with others, the more you become like them. So, choose well the company you keep.

During the time spent with those in your support system, you also make memories linked to positive emotions. As you recall these memories, you allow the same surge of positivity to flood your mind and body, similar to when these events happened. These memories become a source of positivity to turn to when you feel down or distressed.

These bonds offer encouragement and support, ease your pain and loneliness, and provide new perspectives on overcoming problems. The happiness, longevity, and improved mental and physical health you obtain from strong, healthy social connections improve your stress management skills.

It is evident these bonds support stress management, but how? And what can you do to make the most of this stress management opportunity?

HOW SOCIAL SUPPORT RELIEVES STRESS

You're familiar with how the SNS (sympathetic nervous system) triggers the stress response and associated changes in your body. New information shows how social interaction with those in your support system can trigger the PSNS (parasympathetic nervous system) to release the correct hormones establishing a calm state. This was the finding of a research study conducted by the University of Utah in 2014. Researchers determined that social interaction triggers the PSNS to release feel-good hormones. Simultaneously, it also lowers cortisol, which is linked to the stress response.[31]

Except for the drop in stress levels, emotional support is also considered a supporting factor in improving self-esteem. It adds to a sense of autonomy, empowering you to display greater confidence and trust in your ability to overcome challenges.[31]

Are you familiar with the feeling of camaraderie existing amongst friends? Being part of such a bond, a connection to something larger than yourself, adds a sense of security and stability to your life. If this type of connection is absent in your life, there are steps you can take to improve these connections and develop stronger bonds.

BUILDING AND MAINTAINING SOCIAL CONNECTIONS

Strong social connections rely on a two-step approach. You have to expand your network by meeting new people, deciding who you would want to include in your network, and then strengthen your bonds with them. Then, you also need to sustain and strengthen your existing bonds. It means – make time for those you care about, reaching out to them regularly, and making sure you spend time with them. Be there for them when they need you, and create memories together.

EXPANDING YOUR NETWORK

You can only strengthen bonds when you have these connections already established. If your support network lacks these connections, you must meet new people, get to know them better, and decide whether you like them enough to include them in your support network. Remember, not everyone you meet will be someone you want to be part of your support network.

A couple of years ago, I relocated to a new city. It was a major transition in my life as I enjoyed such comfort where I had lived. I was painfully aware that I was leaving behind friends, family, and a warm sense of familiarity. I felt this especially when I got onto the plane with packed bags and thought of all my boxes and belongings, loaded and in transit with the removal company.

Initially, I was on the phone often, checking in with my loved ones at home, but I soon realized that I had to establish a support system where I was. Honestly, there were several failed attempts to make new friends. I attended every social event coworkers invited me to, and sometimes, I met very nice people at these functions. But there were also many times when I didn't click with people.

Yet, I didn't give up. I just cast my net a bit wider. I joined a hiking club and went on trips with these people, making wonderful friends in this group. My new best friend I met in a bookshop. This wonderful little bookshop is a couple of streets away from my apartment. It is such a gem and one of those cute, old-fashioned shops that are becoming really hard to find nowadays.

I met Rodney, the owner, through my regular trips to this shop, and we became friends. Today, Rodney is a dear friend who has played a valuable role in my support network.

Where can you go to meet new friends?

REACH OUT

Making friends will depend on you. You can't sit at home and expect to meet new people. Strangers don't just arrive at your doorstep, strike up a conversation and eventually leave as friends. Also, you can't say that you never meet new people if you don't place yourself in a position to do so.

Go out to places where you can meet others. There are so many places where you'll be able to meet people. Join a club where you'll meet others with interests similar to yours. Volunteer your time to meet others or smile at strangers who may become friends.

MAINTAIN EXISTING BONDS

Are you still attending family dinners, weddings, funerals, or birthday parties? I know some of these events can be morbid, but I've had some of the best catching-up sessions with my cousins, nieces, and nephews at the funerals of uncles and aunts. Family members may stay far away from each other but often will make an effort to attend these events.

Remember to never take the people in your life for granted. Send them a text message asking how they're doing. Or give them a call to tell them you're thinking of them. Stay close to those you care about. It will require effort from your side but it's effort well worth making. These connections and the bonds that they create can be so rewarding.

FIND OTHERS IN SIMILAR SITUATIONS

The challenges you face can be a bond that brings you and others together. As you share the same challenges, you already have a connection point and clarity on what the other person is going through and how to support them.

There is a community hall on my way home from work. One day, I noticed a group of gray-haired men standing outside chatting. There were no more than six or seven. However, as the weeks passed, I noticed the group was getting larger. I got curious and stopped one day to ask them about their meeting. They eagerly told me that they are a group of veterans who all live in the city, and they met weekly to share experiences and offer each other support. This support was initially linked to recovering from their experiences as veterans but has gradually turned into offering support with ordinary challenges too. Being a veteran was what connected them. What are the challenges you're facing that can help you connect with others?

These connections can also develop online. A friend of mine is gluten intolerant and has joined a social media page for people who suffer from celiac disease. She made online connections with people who knew what she was going through. Another friend has extraordinarily curly hair, and she joined a group with other curly-haired women to discuss their curly hair challenges. Apparently, their issues are numerous and important enough to seek support for!

Set aside any assumptions that you need a big, fancy problem before you're allowed to join or create communities of support. Initially, the conversations will start with matters linked to your common interests. Then, naturally, the bonds proceed past just your shared interest.

ASK FOR HELP WHEN NEEDED

Community centers, places of worship, libraries, neighborhood clinics, health centers, or even refugee or immigrant groups can be easy to find today. Identify the obstacles you're facing and the support you need, then identify where you'll find the help you desire. Search your local notice boards and online pages, or even ask where you can find professionals to support you.

REACH OUT, BUT DON'T APPLY ANY PRESSURE

Understand that not everyone will reply to an invitation as you might have hoped. People are busy or under stress. They may not be up to attending to your invitation, or they don't have the time. Don't take others declining your invitations personally. And don't pressure them to accept next time. Rather be flexible and understand they can't make it now, but there is always another time.

Even if you want to discuss something important with someone, first check whether it is a good time for them to listen to you. If not, you risk not getting the attention you deserve and desire. Rather check first and prevent disappointment.

FORGIVE AND FORGIVE AGAIN

OK, you were ignored by someone from whom you would have least expected it. Maybe that person canceled on short notice and didn't explain why.

My mother used to get very upset when this happened to her. Once, she had a lunch date with my aunt, who never showed up. Mom returned home visibly upset. She was fuming for days about what happened and refused to send my aunt a message to find out why it happened. Mom had all the reasons to hold on to her resentment.

Only after two weeks, when she bumped into a mutual friend of hers and my aunt, she heard that my aunt had fallen and broken her hip and was stuck in the hospital. Due to all the drama in my aunt's life, she forgot to let Mom know she won't be there for lunch.

Don't hold grudges. You may never truly know why people stood you up or declined your invitation. Instead, let go, forgive, and move on.

SHOW GRATITUDE

When was the last time you told the people in your life how much they mean to you? Express your appreciation, either verbally or through taking action. Everyone likes to hear they're appreciated, so write that card or send a thank you message.

LISTEN ACTIVELY

To have someone in your life that will support you, you also need to be someone who is willing to help others. So, when people need your support, have to vent about something, or need a shoulder to cry on, be that person. Listen when they speak, show you understand, and ensure the other person feels heard.

IDENTIFY BONDS THAT DON'T SUPPORT YOUR GOALS

Not all relationships serve you. Getting trapped in a relationship where you feel used or one that leaves you drained can be easy. Keep in mind that the people you surround yourself with will have an impact on your life. So, be discerning about whom you keep around. If a friendship is toxic, it will keep you locked in the stress response.

Essentially the level of success you'll enjoy from your bonds and increasing their strength depends on how well you can communicate.

STEPS TO IMPROVE YOUR COMMUNICATION

It can be easy to limit communication to merely saying what you want, but effective communication depends on much more than that. Only a small segment of communication depends on the spoken word; a lot more is communicated through tone, non-verbal sounds, gestures, expressions, and body language. Only through active listening will you become aware of all these aspects of communication and how you'll be able to gather the entirety of what is being said to you.

So, if you want to improve your relationships by improving communication, you must become an active listener. Without an active listener, any communication will be a monologue.

SUCCESS IN THE MANNER YOU EXPRESS YOURSELF

At the end of this section, you'll know what it entails to be a great listener, but you have no certainty that the person you're talking to possesses these skills or, if they do, is applying them while you speak. Hence, keeping communication clear and concise will be to your favor.

Oversharing information can distract the message you want to convey. That said, you need to be sure that the other person understands the context of your message. A fine line, right? Indeed it is, and it is a balance you can find by reading your audience. Does the listener seem engaged? Are they maintaining eye contact? Are there any distractions you're competing against? What does their body language express?

Some conversations are harder to have than others. Just think how hard it can be to ask for an increase or a promotion. Yet, difficult conversations are part of life, and your success and happiness may depend on these conversations.

Regarding these conversations, you must be sure you've chosen the right timing. There shouldn't be distractions keeping the other person from giving their full attention. Nor should you have to compete against time. The last thing you want to do is to create animosity, so stick to I-statements. For example, don't say, "You always treat me like dirt!" Rather opt for the kinder version of, "I often feel undervalued in your presence."

Consider your last difficult conversation. How did it work out for you? Did you achieve the outcome you desired? If not, can you identify your mistakes in communicating your message?

SUCCESSFUL COMMUNICATION BY LISTENING ACTIVELY

I encourage you to take the following test. Over the next few days, note where your mind wanders when someone is talking to you. Determine whether you listen to the end of what they're saying or if your mind wanders in all directions to determine the best way to respond to a fragment of their message you caught early on.

Don't be too hard on yourself if you are guilty of this. It just means that you're just like many others. That's right. We tend to be so quick to compose an answer to justify or defend ourselves that we miss most of what is being said.

A far better approach is to wait until the end, pause to think about your answer, and then reply based on everything you've heard.

By maintaining eye contact, you convey to the speaker that you're still listening. Simply showing that they have your full attention can defuse any negative emotions linked to harder conversations. But it is also active listening that will strengthen the bonds between you and others.

Keep your body language open. Having your hands on your lap is a perfect way to show that you're receiving information. You can also show interest by asking questions to clarify matters you're unsure of or by repeating what you've heard them say to be sure you got the message they wanted to convey.

Are you aware of your body gestures, facial expressions, and the non-verbal sounds you make while listening?

Years ago, as a student, I was assigned a mentor to guide me in writing a thesis. I had to visit the professor's office for bi-weekly meetings as predetermined by the university. I dreaded every meeting. The professor would hardly ever engage with what I was saying. He would stare in my direction, but I always felt that he was lost, looking at something behind me. Whenever he replied, it wasn't directly addressing my concerns. It was hard for me as a young student to succeed in my academic career with the type of support I had to rely on.

One morning I arrived for another dreaded meeting, and a new professor was in the chair on the other side of the desk. I discovered that my mentor had fallen ill. I wasn't bothered with the details of his illness but I did take delight in learning that he was booked off for the rest of the year, and in front of me was my new mentor!

My new mentor was always engaged in every conversation. He was open to what I said, looked me in the eyes as I spoke, and asked many questions to ensure he understood what I meant so he could advise me accurately. He would nod, while his "aha," at the right moments, ensured that he was following every word I said. We formed a strong bond and my whole academic experience shifted simply because of his listening and communication skills.

GETTING BETTER AT MINDFUL COMMUNICATIONS

Mindful communication means that you're present and remain aware of all that is said. It is an approach ensuring more effective communication.

A lot can be said about mindful communication, and there is a lot you can learn if you want to become a master in this skill. But for now, I want to focus on these two mistakes so commonly made, which you can improve on right away.

REFRAIN FROM JUDGING

"You know, Jimmy just has to look at me in a certain way, and then I know he will ask for more money. It is when I immediately switch off. I just can't listen to it all anymore," John, a former colleague, was livid as his son only contacts them when he is broke.

Or that was at least how John perceived the matter.

It is so easy to make judgment calls about what will be said early on and then to "switch off" as John did.

Are you guilty of listening only for the first few seconds, and your mind drifts and seeks ways to address the matter? Sure, like John, you have people who regularly repeat the same stories or patterns, but copying John's approach won't serve your bonds.

Rather focus on remaining present to the end. Then you can reply with a well-structured answer addressing every aspect of what is being said.

John's usual reply to Jimmy would be, "How much do you need?" Upon which Jimmy would give an embarrassed laugh and make his number. I could see John didn't like seeing his son only when he needed to make a cash withdrawal. So, we discussed this pattern thoroughly.

Finally, John decided to listen to the very end of Jimmy's story rather than make a judgment call early on. It was quite an emotional moment when John walked into my office the next day.

"Jimmy was here yesterday," he started.

"Oh, OK," I replied.

"He's part of a band, ya know? He told me all about a tour that he and his band are planning."

"And?" I wanted to know.

"And that was it. He didn't ask for money. I didn't offer. I just listened to everything he said. I barely knew anything about his music or his passion for it and I definitely didn't know that the money I had been giving him meant that he could pursue this passion instead of having to give it all up and take a boring job, just for the sake of money." John was so proud and he saw so much purpose in what he'd been inadvertently supporting all this time. It was also clear that he regretted missing out on so many of the conversations his son had with him over the past couple of years.

What are you missing out on just because you jump to judgment prematurely?

DON'T DRAW COMPARISONS

"I made a huge mistake. I don't know how I am going to fix it."

My sister was close to tears as she expanded on an event that had taken place between herself and her daughter the previous day. Her daughter shared something personal with her, something that would take a lot of guts for any teenage girl to tell her mom. However, instead of responding with empathy and understanding, my sister replied, "You're just like your father."

This wouldn't have been an insult if my sister's ex-husband was a man to be proud of, but he wasn't. He failed his wife and daughter miserably when he walked out years ago, leaving the two to take care of themselves. While it is only natural for my niece to have certain features of her dad as they share the same genetics, this comparison is insulting because of what he did to them.

For the sake of your own important connections, refrain from making the same mistake. It's rarely, if ever, helpful to compare anyone with others or one situation with another. Instead, protect your relationships through more mindful communication.

Similarly, as we know that it's impossible to accurately read another person's mind, never assume you know what the other person will say. Or that your listeners will automatically understand what you mean. Always focus on every aspect of communication to ensure you accurately interpret what the other person is talking about and communicate with clarity to give listeners accurate insight into your mind.

Talking is so easy it encourages a disregard for the importance of effective communication. Yet, effective communication can be challenging. By investing a little effort, you can significantly improve your communication, making your efforts to establish and maintain strong bonds that much more successful. These healthy bonds will be a helpful aid in your stress management practices. In the next chapter, I want you to shift your perspective from outside to within again. Here our focus is on the vagus nerve, the connection bringing together so many aspects of your existence. It is a vital element to explore on your stress management journey. So, let's move on, as I am sure you're keen to take the final steps toward recovery and gaining control over stress in your life.

To Do List For Less Stress:

Make friends

Forgive everyone

Listen carefully

Don't judge

Don't compare

Communicate

and above all ...

Be grateful

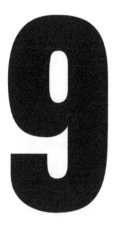

9

THE
HARMONY
HIGHWAY

**Your Vagus Nerve And
Why It's So Spectacular!**

*The vagus nerve is involved in nearly every
physiological action in the human body and
harnessing its power can have an immediate
and dramatic impact on your well-being.*

– Suzanne Krowiak[32]

"Bless you!" is probably the most common response to an event that indicates your vagus nerve is in excellent working order. Yes, sneezing is a reaction we can thank the vagus nerve for.

Similarly, swallowing, breathing, vomiting, heart rate, and digestion are all functions that originate in the vagus nerve.

WHAT IS THE VAGUS NERVE?

The vagus nerve is also known as the pneumogastric (*pneu-mo-gas-tric*) nerve and is one of 12 cranial nerves. Cranial nerves emerge directly from the brain rather than from the spinal cord. They control a wide range of functions, including vision, hearing, smell, taste, movement of the eyes, face, and tongue, and swallowing. Each of the cranial nerves is named according to its function. For example, the olfactory nerve is responsible for smell. The facial nerve manages your facial muscles and the optical nerve is in charge of your vision.

The vagus nerve is the longest of the cranial nerves with the broadest range of functions. It begins in the brainstem and reaches all the way down your neck and deep into your chest and abdomen. It is the critical link between the gut and the brain and the foundation of the brain-gut axis.

You may have never even heard of this nerve before but that hasn't stopped it from working for your entire life on your heart rate, managing your blood pressure, controlling your lungs, digestion, speech, taste and the pain sensations in your chest.

The nerve is considered a mixed nerve because it carries both somatic and visceral information. The somatic component carries information from the body to the brain about voluntary movements such as swallowing and talking. The visceral component is responsible for involuntary functions such as heart rate, blood pressure and digestion.

This life force engine is humming away inside of you and performs several functions within your autonomic nervous system which, in turn, is responsible for actions sustaining your overall wellness. The vagus nerve is an incredibly important member of the team of crucial nerves and structures that make up your nervous system.

But, of course, it is hidden and often remains unknown, so it is regularly underused in attempts to establish effective stress management. But, by the end of this chapter, you'll be familiar with a range of easy steps you can use to manipulate this system to your benefit, quickly restoring a state of inner peace and calm.

THE CONNECTION BETWEEN THE VAGUS NERVE AND THE NERVOUS SYSTEM

You're taking a stroll in the park and notice a couple of kids kicking a ball. You enjoy the moment, watching the kids having fun, laughing, and fooling around. It is a happy moment, but then it all goes sour. One kid kicks the ball out of the play area. His teammates are clearly upset, for they've lost the match. They call him *stupid* and push him around. You can hear by what they shout that they'll never pick him for their team again. He walks away with his shoulders and head hung low. You feel his pain and want to rush to tell him *it is okay*. That he is better than what his teammates say and shouldn't base his self-worth on the opinion of others, but you don't. You're a stranger; he is a kid, and you don't feel it would be appropriate. But still long after he is out of sight, you feel his pain.

♥ THE LOVE NERVE

The ability to feel empathy toward another is, in part, thanks to the vagus nerve. It is connected to regions of the brain involved in emotional processing and social cognition. As such, it has occasionally referred to as the love nerve. It plays an important role in emotional regulation and is an undeniable part of stress regulation. It is the nerve that helps you to maintain a sense of calm even when you're in a stressful situation. It helps you return to a state of rest and digest[34] also known as the parasympathetic response – a counterbalance to the "fight or flight" response activated during stressful situations.

Instead, when the vagus nerve is activated, your heart rate lowers, your blood pressure decreases, and a sense of relaxation is restored. This helps to manage the physiological effects of stress and return the body to a calmer state.

GUT FEELING

Remember the ENS? The enteric nervous system. We've discussed this earlier. It's sometimes considered the second brain and it refers to the complex network of neurons located in the 'gut'. The ENS can communicate with the central nervous system, including the brain, and it does so through the vagus nerve.

This is where 'gut feelings' originate. A gut feeling can occur when your brain perceives a sense of fear. Through the link that your vagus nerve creates between your brain and your gut, your brain sends communication about fear, anxiety, and distress to the gut, causing discomfort. The vagus nerve carries these signals bi-directionally, allowing the gut to send information to the brain and vice versa. Discomfort in your gut may be an indication that your brain has detected something disturbing. Fear could be present in your mind, but you feel it in your gut – a gut feeling.

THE BRIDGE CONNECTING MIND AND BODY

The vagus nerve is a vital connector between the mind and body. It is the nerve that can allow us to alternate between being immersed in the stress response and entering a state of calm. This process tended to happen naturally for our caveman, but now life is different. Modern-day threats pose different challenges, and we've explored that alternating between the stress response and a state of calm is no longer so easy and doesn't occur as autonomously as we might like. This change is increasing the importance of understanding and improving the works of the vagus nerve.

Thankfully, it's entirely possible to condition your vagus nerve to function more effectively, ensuring a state of calm and restoring your mind and body's resting state. Improving the functioning of your vagus nerve will improve your response to stress and your ability to manage it effectively.

Whilst many of the steps discussed in this book will contribute positively to your vagus nerve's condition, there are several specific steps you can take to directly improve this vital function.

TECHNIQUES TO IMPROVE HOW YOUR VAGUS NERVE RESPONDS

The mind-body connection enables you to gain control over your vagus nerve through specific exercise and breathing combinations.

A BASIC TECHNIQUE

Let's start with the most straightforward step to improve this connection. The movements captured under the exercise are easy. They're an effective way to increase awareness of your body and what is happening internally. This is a great way to begin to activate the vagus nerve and improve its stimulation to regulate your stress response.

1. Get comfortable on your back with your hands behind your head.

2. Interweave your fingers.

3. Start by looking straight ahead of you at the ceiling above.

4. Without moving your head, look as far as possible to the right.

5. Hold this position until you spontaneously yawn or swallow.

6. Only then can you return to the starting position, looking straight ahead.

7. Repeat the exercise, looking to the other side until your body spontaneously yawns or swallows.

What has just happened? By moving your eyes in this manner, you actively connect the eight suboccipital (*sub-oc-cip-i-tal*) muscles with those responsible for moving your eyes. The suboccipital muscles are located in four groups at the back of your neck in the same area where your vagus nerve is connected and their proximity allows for potential interactions and influences between the two. This is one very simple way to activate the vagus nerve to establish a state of greater calm.[34].

THE HALF SALAMANDER EXERCISE

This exercise can be done seated, so you can activate it anywhere you find yourself needing to activate your vagus nerve to lower your stress levels. This exercise is highly effective in activating the vagus nerve. So, try it once you're comfortable with the previously mentioned technique.

1. Keep your head straight while looking to the right as far as possible.

2. Then tilt your head to the right toward your shoulder while maintaining your view.

3. Hold this position for a minute.

4. Bring back your eyes and head to the center, a neutral state ahead of you.

5. Look to the left while holding your head straight before tilting your head toward your left shoulder.

6. Hold this position again for a minute before returning to your neutral state, looking right ahead. As the vagus nerve plays a pivotal role in breathing, you can also use your body to activate the vagus nerve through breathing exercises.

The eye movements this activity is based upon have been linked to overall brain activation and positive effects on the autonomic nervous system. Tilting your head to the side while maintaining your gaze can stretch and engage the muscles and tissues in your neck and upper body. This movement can help release tension, promote blood flow, and influence the activity of nerves, including those connected to the vagus nerve.

BREATHING EXERCISES THAT ACTIVATE THE VAGUS NERVE

Several exercises can help activate the vagus nerve, allowing it to respond better to stress.

GARGLING, SINGING, HUMMING, AND CHANTING

One of my favorite childhood memories is sitting around the campfire, listening to my grandpa's ghost stories. He was an amazing storyteller and would keep the attention of his grandchildren, all staring at him with wide eyes as he shared colorful versions of scary tales night after night. I remembered how the characters in his gripping tales would often whistle or sing when they got scared, and I never understood why. Now I know any action causing vibration in the throat can help to wake up the vagus nerve. Humming and singing, or even gargling, can do the same trick.

When you're ready to activate these same benefits for yourself, find a quiet spot where you can chant the word *ohm* several times. Yes, this is the sound often associated with meditation or spiritual practice. It is said to have calming and centering effects on the mind and body, helping to induce a state of relaxation, focus, and spiritual connection.

Like gargling and humming, laughter also generates positive vibrations in your body. Is there a better way than laughter to create vibrations in your body? If there is, I'm yet to find out. So, let out the raucous, belly laughter. This will always lift your mood, and boost your immune system too!

BELLY BREATHING

Early on, I mentioned belly breathing as a method to induce a state of calm by triggering the PSNS. Belly breathing is a technique where you deliberately breathe so deeply that your diaphragm moves up and down in conjunction with the chest cavity expansion. You can succeed with this breathing exercise in several ways, and while any version will do, I recommend the steps below.

1. Place one hand on your stomach and the other on your chest.

2. Take a deep breath and feel how your chest cavity expands, pushing your hand up before the diaphragm pushes your belly up to make room for your chest cavity to expand.

3. While taking these deep breaths, your heart rate slows, and your blood pressure drops simultaneously.

Other simple tricks are to make your exhales a bit longer than your inhales. By exhaling longer than you inhale, your body immediately shifts into a state of relaxation. Try it now. Inhale for four counts, hold your breath, and exhale for six counts. Repeat a few times and see how well it works.

STIMULATING THE DIVING REFLEX

Have you ever felt emotionally overwhelmed? I imagine so. Have you ever felt as though you wanted to dive into a cold ocean, river or pool to cool down your turbulent emotions?

By immersing in cold water you would activate the vagus nerve by stimulating the diving reflex through exposure to the cold. The diving reflex is a physiological response that occurs when the body is exposed to cold water, particularly on the face and neck.

Excusing yourself from an intense meeting to hop into a pool is not always a practical solution. Thankfully, just splashing your face with cold water will have a similar effect. You can also rub an ice cube on your face for instant improvement. The cold exposure will immediately slow your heart rate, relax your body, and cause your anxiety to plummet.

FOOT RUBS

A foot massage is one of my favorite ways to relax and even though it's not directly linked to activating the vagus nerve, it can promote a feeling of overall well–being and therefore influence the vagal tone. A higher vagal tone is generally associated with greater parasympathetic activity and better regulation of bodily functions. It indicates a more adaptive stress response, improved cardiovascular health, enhanced digestion, lower inflammation, and better emotional well–being. So whether it's a foot rub, a sauna or a night at a comedy show, lifting your vagal tone should be the intention behind as many daily activities as possible.

None of these techniques require much time nor are they hard to do, yet they can improve your stress levels immediately. By practicing these techniques, you'll become more comfortable with them and develop greater control over your vagus nerve and the corresponding benefits that produces. Your Workbook has an activity that shows you how to incorporate one or many of these exercises into your regular routine.

Before we meet each other in the very last chapter of this book, where I will review some of the vital information we've shared, I want to expand on one more technique you can apply to control how your body responds to stress. *Forest bathing* is a well-known Japanese practice used to restore a state of mental and emotional calm, extending to physical calmness and relaxation also.

FOREST BATHING

Earlier on, I mentioned the benefit of spending time in green spaces, but there is more to say about this ancient practice. Forest bathing doesn't involve a bath but it's more than merely going for a stroll in the forest. It's a mindfulness practice, allowing yourself to become immersed in the tranquility of your settings. Forest 'bathing' means to spend time in green spaces, like a forest, and to shift your focus to the sights, sounds, and scents surrounding you. The technique forces you into a greater state of mindfulness. By getting swept away by your surroundings, you enjoy an emotional calm, forcing your brain to stop ruminating, worrying, or anticipating what will happen next.

Remember, stress is nestled in the past or future, but the present moment can be a stress-free gift. You can become entirely relaxed by spending time in an environment where you can immerse yourself in a stress-free state.

Forest bathing is an effective method to enjoy a greater sense of calm and it is backed by scientific research. Researchers found that forest therapy reduces cortisol levels, causes blood pressure to drop, and even improves blood sugar levels[35].

We have covered a lot of ground so far. You've absorbed a lot of vital information, several strategies and tips, all with potentially life-changing benefits and the ability to improve your well-being.

In the next chapter, I'll sort and summarize this information for you to ensure you leave our time together with clarity and practical solutions for effectively managing stress in your life.

10

MAKE IT
ALL HAPPEN

How You Can Use These Tools
In Real Life

*Knowledge is useless without
consistent application.*

– Julian Hall[36]

Years ago, I was very passionate about photography. I still think it is a wonderful art form, but I no longer find myself behind the camera. When I began, I was very excited and I made a few impulsive and expensive purchases in this hyped state. This included a beautiful camera and state-of-the-art photo editing software. However, photography was merely a hobby, and whenever work got very busy, there was often limited time to invest in my hobby. I had all the necessary tools to hone my craft, and then some, but I never did. I never fully understood the camera's function or how to use the software effectively. Both ended up barely being used. While I could sell the camera and get some of my money back, the software became a loss I had to write off. If I had invested more time in understanding how these tools worked, I would've been able to create visual masterpieces, but I never did. I lost the opportunity of learning a new skill, expanding my knowledge base, and creating beauty, soothing to the eye and the soul, because I failed to invest time in familiarizing myself with the tools I possessed.

The same is true when it comes to the nervous system. It is a wonderous, miraculous system, controlling every aspect of your life and existence, your well-being, and the state of the platform you build your future upon. Yet, it is a system most are unaware of and rarely bother to explore, or get familiar with. As your nervous system is out of sight, it can also remain out of mind. That's understandable. You can see your hand and be aware of its functioning, but the nervous system is unseen and, therefore, quickly forgotten. So, instead of caring for it, you forget its far-reaching influence on your existence and what a powerful resource it is.

It's my intention that you don't do that. I would love to think that the information you've gathered here will not just heighten your awareness of the role your nervous system plays in your life but that you will take a very active role in maintaining a healthy, stable nervous system that supports your best existence.

Your body and health are not a fad or a hobby, like my photography. They are the basis upon which you create the quality of your life. The information you now have gives you the ability to dramatically improve the quality of your body, your health and your life. In this chapter, I'll present this information so that you have every chance to make this new awareness become a consistent theme in your decisions and actions.

YOUR PERSONAL STRESSORS AND TRIGGERS

Have you been able to pinpoint the stressors in your life? Knowing the triggers causing your stress is an important step to utilizing your new understanding of the nervous system. Some very common life stressors are:

- Health concerns

- The state of your relationships

- Financial stress

- Life changes

- Emotional problems

- Personal beliefs can trigger stress. Some examples of such beliefs are beliefs related to religion, politics, or beliefs linked to your value system. The latter occurs when your values conflict with the views of others or those in your environment.

- When you're discriminated against or even just witnessing discrimination.

- Environmental factors, like disasters, poverty, or oppression.

- Your career can trigger stress in several ways.

In the exercise below, you'll be invited to identify your stressors as part of building a plan for your nervous system regulation. For now, it's enough to contemplate the list above and give some thought to your own version of these and other stressors more specific to your circumstances. Later in this chapter, you'll see how you can use the stressors you've identified in a written Workbook activity.

DEVELOPING YOUR PERSONALIZED NERVOUS SYSTEM REGULATION PLAN

The value of this book is fully realized through taking action, but sometimes the gap between understanding what to do and doing it can be wide and hard to cross. Even now, you've enriched your mind with a wealth of knowledge about your nervous system and the many steps you can take to achieve your desired outcome. However, you may appreciate some direction toward your first step on your recovery journey.

Allow the following steps to guide you, to be your bridge across the gap that may appear hard to cross.

STEP 1: IDENTIFY THE PROBLEM YOU'RE FACING

How have you ended up with this book in your hands? What was the problem that became the catalyst for your initial interest? Can you identify, acknowledge, and describe your personal situation? If you can, you know where you are. That's the first of three aspects of a well-planned journey, whether that journey is a cross-country trip or traveling to your local convenience store or, indeed, healing your nervous system.

First, you need to know where you are, then where you're going, and the most efficient route between these points. So, before proceeding, describe your current situation in detail. Identify your stressors, and understand their impact on your life.

 This exercise is repeated in your Workbook with space to document the process and prompts to help you along.

Can you avoid the stressors causing you concern? Is it possible to avoid certain situations, events, or people you know cause your stress levels to spike? That's not always going to be possible. So, thankfully, this book offers you tools that allow you to enter stressful situations with calmness and confidence.

STEP 2: TAKING CARE OF YOUR "VEHICLE"

In this case, your vehicle is your body and mind. Nutrition, exercise, quality sleep, and sufficient relaxation ensure your body is a safe and reliable vehicle to get you where you need to go without breaking down. I've shared many techniques and strategies, and the temptation may be to take on as many as you can carry, but refrain. Taking on too many changes at a time will provide its own stress and overwhelm. Instead, stick to small but persistent changes. This is how you create transformation.

 In your Workbook, you'll see the techniques available to you and you'll be prompted to find room in your life for the ones that fit your circumstances and your current needs.

STEP 3: ADDRESS YOUR EMOTIONS

Could you describe your current emotional state? If you never have to or even want to articulate how you feel, your emotions will remain largely unknown. If so, it's hard for you to understand what's happening and almost impossible for anyone to help you make sense of what you're experiencing. You create an extra, unnecessary burden for yourself by just putting up with the emotions that arrive instead of acknowledging them, describing them, perhaps sharing them with others and actively seeking a resolution to the ones that don't serve you. Shakespeare said: "Give sorrow words; the grief that does not speak knits up the o-er wrought heart and bids it break."[37]. I think what he means is "Express your sorrow through words; if your grief remains unspoken, it tightens your burdened heart and eventually causes it to break."

In your Workbook there is an exercise that invites you to express yourself. It can remain strictly private if you choose but you may decide to share it with those in your support network (Chapter 8). You may even take these words to your spiritual practice and pray over them. These expressions may form the basis of your meditation, mindful movement, breathing exercises, or other techniques we've discussed.

I know you'll find this a powerful exercise, particularly if you're not in the habit of sharing your thoughts or emotions freely.

STEP 4: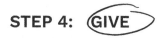

What you gain from giving is an emotional surge equaled by few other actions. It could be your time or service, your money, your possessions or anything of value. Giving brings a sense of purpose, pleasure, value, gratitude, belonging and accomplishment. Can you volunteer? How can you offer your services and contribute to the life of another? Can you offer your experience and advice on a topic or a cause? Can you help your neighbor? Can you take the clothes you no longer wear to the local thrift store? Can you join a movement, help a cause or even start one yourself?

 "You can never go broke giving money away" 99
— J. Paul Getty.

If you're seeking circuit-breaking stress relief, give. Put yourself in the way of people who need help. You'll quickly discover two things: (1) Your own value to others; and (2) the relative insignificance of your own problems.

These four steps, in combination with the other techniques and strategies I've shared with you, form the basis of your nervous system regulation plan. Make sure you visit the Workbook to see how these steps can happen in real life.

Applying Stress Management Techniques In Real-Life Situations

Once you have your plan has been created and it's being implemented, you'll be taking proactive steps to protect your mental, emotional, and physical health from exposure to stress. That said, life will still present innumerable challenges, but you will be infinitely better equipped to handle them when they arise. Below are some examples where your stress management skills may be required.

STRESS MANAGEMENT AT HOME

Home is supposed to be your safe haven, a place where you can relax and recuperate. Yet, life isn't always as we expect it to be. Stressors can still appear at home, despite being the place where you seek refuge.

1. Even at home, especially at home, speak up for yourself. Be heard and state what you need. Let others know how you expect to be treated, where your boundaries lie and what you simply won't tolerate. The best

way to demonstrate your preferences is to lead by example. Respect, for example, cannot be expected unless it is first shown.

2. If your home environment presents problems that cause stress levels to spike, you need to take active steps toward solving those problems, with a sense of urgency about it. Don't just build your resilience so that you're comfortable with bad situations. Seek solutions instead. For example, if money is constantly the source of stress, don't allow a lack of any budgetary control to continually magnify your financial weakness. Sit down, open your computer, create a spreadsheet and work out where the money is going and then start plugging those financial holes. If the problem is illness, turn the TV off and research the issue. Examine your diet. Be honest about your exercise routine or complete lack of it. No more complaining. Start aiming at solutions instead.

3. Stress manages to accumulate rapidly in chaotic environments. A lot of the stress you experience can dissipate once you get organized in every aspect of life. This will include your personal and shared spaces and time management and planning. Get a diary. Plan out your days. Clear out the closets. Get rid of everything in the cupboards past the 'best before' date. Start tidying it all up and bask in the peacefulness of good order.

4. Sometimes the best thing you can do to enjoy instant relief is to step into a safe space. Do you have a room at home where you can be alone and dedicate time to self-care? If not, create a plan for creating such a space in your home. It can be a shed, a spare bedroom or even just the living room for one hour a day when everyone knows that this is *your time* without any interruptions.

STRESS MANAGEMENT IN YOUR RELATIONSHIPS

Just because you care deeply for another doesn't mean the relationship will be stress-free.

1. Sometimes the stress that occurs in relationships can be the most intense and impactful of all. The communications between partners, friends and family can be fraught with challenges, past wounds and the

fear of negative consequences. Some of your most productive stress management activities will be improving the communication in such relationships. This could mean some deep and personal therapeutic work. It will almost definitely involve reading some new, helpful books, listening to good podcasts and learning new skills. If you're not active in this area of growth, you can expect the stress to remain. Make it a priority to enhance your relationships through improved communication. It's a necessity.

2. We so often complain or confront something that we suspect is the right thing to target when the reality is that the source of our stress is buried way beneath the apparent problem. If you've been attempting to resolve something for weeks, months or even years, perhaps it's time to pause and think deeply about what the real problem is. If the problem is persistent dispute much arguing and frustration, chances are the problem is you and chances are also good that it's a problem that originated in your childhood. Pause, get clear on what's triggering all of this upset and go to work on the real cause. Not the people around you that you're blaming for it.

3. Even in the closest, healthiest relationships, it is so important to set time apart for yourself, to spend alone, investing in your well-being.

4. If your communication skills appear to be at the center of many of your stressors, I think my best advice has to be – improve your communication skills. Return to chapter eight and make that your focus until the stress starts to dissolve.

STRESS MANAGEMENT AT WORK

The office environment can quickly turn into a hostile space where an unhealthy stress level constantly exists. I have four tips for effective stress management in this more formal environment.

1. Be sure to know what is expected from you. This may often relate to your workload and the expectations of your co-workers. Once you have gained clarity on this, once you know what you're expected to deliver

and what you're not willing to commit to, communicate this effectively to avoid friction or confrontation later.

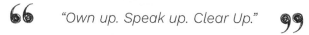 *"Own up. Speak up. Clear Up."*

2. Contrary to old beliefs, multitasking isn't the special domain of the hyper-productive. Far from it. It's a stress-inducing approach that diminishes productivity. Don't get caught in the trap of thinking that looking busy makes you more important. To divide is not to conquer. To focus is what will help you achieve your best results.

3. Don't let conflict erupt. Particularly when you can see it coming from a mile away. You've been around long enough to know the patterns. When you see it approaching, when Gary sparks up another debate in the weekly meeting, step in and take action. It is easier to prevent damage from occurring, even if it does lead to mild confrontations, than having to mop up after things are left to spin out of control.

4. Get comfortable. Don't sit on that hard chair for 4 hours and eat lunch at your desk and then walk for miles to the train in your work shoes and then stand for an hour amongst the other commuters. You know how it's going to feel to do all those things. You did it yesterday, and you were miserable. Get a comfy seat, take a break for lunch, sit outside in the sun, bring your trainers to work so you can wear them on the walk home. Be smart. You deserve to feel good. It will cascade into every decision your make and every interaction you have with others. Others deserve to benefit from you feeling good for the sake of their own stress levels.

5. It is a lot of information, but the most important underlying factor sustaining your stress management plan at work is to get comfortable. Being in discomfort for extended periods will increase your stress levels, and you'll be better off avoiding this risk. Invest in an ergonomically-friendly chair and desk, and do what is necessary to prevent tension build-up due to discomfort.

TROUBLESHOOTING

Even though you may have a better understanding of how to manage stress, interpreting that as to mean that you can now embrace more stress is not how to view this. It still remains wise to avoid stress where possible, even if you've got a solution for when it does occur.

When situations get heated, wherever possible, step away. Even though you are well-equipped to compose yourself through the exercises you're now familiar with, gain distance between yourself and your stressor instead. After all, the stress response is called the fight or flight response, and it isn't necessary to always opt to fight your way to safety. Sure, there are benefits to confronting your obstacles, but sometimes the outcome of such friction is just not worth sacrificing your sanity.

THE BENEFITS OF EFFECTIVE NERVOUS SYSTEM REGULATION TECHNIQUES

In case you've gotten this far and are still wondering, below you'll see the benefits you can expect from employing these nervous system regulation tools. I mean, you picked up this book for a reason. Perhaps there was a need, some pain, maybe the discomfort of unwanted experiences in your life, and you knew you needed to find a solution. Well, these are the benefits you can expect by implementing the ideas we've now shared:

- A stress level that is both lower and easier to manage

- Falling asleep quickly and enjoying sufficient hours of uninterrupted sleep.

- Improved holistic health and well being

- More meaningful relationships that enrich your life

- Clear focus and lasting concentration that enhances your productivity

- Enjoying life with increased ease and comfort

Are these the things you're seeking? Even if the exact need in your mind isn't listed in specific words, it will fall under one of the categories above. That is a promise I confidently make; as you've seen, the nervous system impacts every aspect of your life, and improving the environment and conditions this system operates in, is bound to bring improvement in every part of your being. You'll gain instant relief and enjoy lasting results through sustained action, applying the shared strategies and tips.

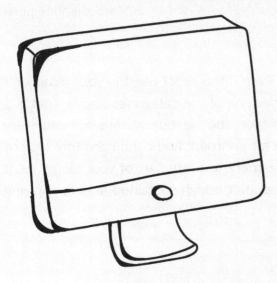

IN 90 SECONDS YOU CAN MAKE A HUGE DIFFERENCE

If you feel we've deserved it, please take a moment to leave a review on Amazon.

Your feedback means the world to us. It helps us to improve and it means better learning experiences for all our readers.

We'd be so grateful to you for your review!

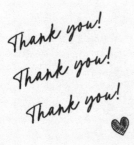

Thank you!
Thank you!
Thank you!

REFERENCES

1. Patterson, E. (2022, September 5). *Stress facts, statistics and trends*. The Recovery Village. https://www.therecoveryvillage.com/mental-health/stress/stress-statistics/#:~:text=About%2033%20percent%20of%20people

2. *Top 25 tools quotes*. (n.d.). A-Z Quotes. https://www.azquotes.com/quotes/topics/tools.html

3. *Brains and nerves*. (n.d.). DK Find Out! https://www.dkfindout.com/us/human-body/brain-and-nerves/

4. Cirino, E. (2019, August 5). *11 Fun facts about the nervous system*. Healthline. https://www.healthline.com/health/fun-facts-about-the-nervous-system#1

5. Salzman, D. (2023). amygdala | Definition, Function, Location, & Facts. In *Encyclopædia Britannica*. https://www.britannica.com/science/amygdala

6. Mani, M. (2019, January 21). *37 Relaxing quotes to help You destress (With beautiful nature images)*. Out of Stress. https://www.outofstress.com/relaxing-quotes-to-destress/

7. Grujicic, R. (2023, April 11). *Sympathetic nervous system*. Kenhub. https://www.kenhub.com/en/library/anatomy/sympathetic-nervous-system

8. Breit, S., Kupferberg, A., Rogler, G., & Hasler, G. (2018). Vagus Nerve as Modulator of the Brain–Gut Axis in Psychiatric and Inflammatory Disorders. *Frontiers in Psychiatry*, 9(44). https://doi.org/10.3389/fpsyt.2018.00044

9. Gerten, K. (2021, June 2). *It's survival. 13 Quotes on trauma & healing*. Youth Dynamics | Mental Health Care for Montana Kids. https://www.youthdynamics.org/its-survival-13-quotes-on-trauma-healing/

10. Lebow, H. I. (2023, January 21). *How does your body remember trauma?* Psych Central. https://psychcentral.com/health/how-your-body-remembers-trauma#next-steps

11. *Pema Chödrön Quote: "Meditation practice isn't about trying to throw ourselves away and become something better. It's about befriending who w…"* (n.d.). Quote Fancy. https://quotefancy.com/quote/887404/Pema-Ch-dr-n-Meditation-practice-isn-t-about-trying-to-throw-ourselves-away-and-become

12.   Better Help Editorial Team. (2023, February 23). *What is the mind-body connection?* Better Help. https://www.betterhelp.com/advice/general/what-is-the-mind-body-connection/

13.   Russo, M. A., Santarelli, D. M., & O'Rourke, D. (2017). The physiological effects of slow breathing in the healthy human. *Breathe, 13*(4), 298–309. https://doi.org/10.1183/20734735.009817

14.   Nunez, K. (2020, August 10). *The benefits of progressive muscle relaxation and how to do it.* Healthline. https://www.healthline.com/health/progressive-muscle-relaxation#about-pmr

15.   Davenport, B. (2022, October 22). *37 Quotes on breathing for a calm and mindful day.* Mindful Zen. https://mindfulzen.co/quotes-breathing/

16.   McGonigal, K. (2020, January 6). *Five surprising ways exercise changes your brain.* Greater Good. https://greatergood.berkeley.edu/article/item/five_surprising_ways_exercise_changes_your_brain

17.   Mosley, B. L. (2022, September 29). *19 Gut health quotes & sayings 2023* . Gut Health Improvement. https://guthealthimprovement.com/gut-health-quotes/

18.   Watson, S. (2020, April 1). *How long does it take to digest food? All about digestion.* Healthline. https://www.healthline.com/health/how-long-does-it-take-to-digest-food#How-long-it-takes-to-digest-food

19.   Cleveland Clinic. (2022, April 21). *Ghrelin.* Cleveland Clinic. https://my.clevelandclinic.org/health/body/22804-ghrelin

20.   Johns Hopkins Medicine. (n.d.). *The brain-gut connection.* John Hopkins Medicine. https://www.hopkinsmedicine.org/health/wellness-and-prevention/the-brain-gut-connection

21.   Carpenter, S. (2012). *That gut feeling.* APA. https://www.apa.org/monitor/2012/09/gut-feeling#:~:text=Gut%20bacteria%20also%20produce%20hundreds

22.   OmegaQuant. (2018, September 25). *How omega-3s might help break the vicious cycle of anxiety.* OmegaQuant. https://omegaquant.com/how-omega-3s-might-help-break-the-vicious-cycle-of-anxiety/

23.   OmegaQuant. (2021, June 3). *Can omega-3 reduce stress?* OmegaQuant. https://omegaquant.com/can-omega-3-reduce-stress/

24.   *3 Ways that protein helps manage stress and anxiety.* (n.d.). Axiom Foods. https://axiomfoods.com/3-ways-that-protein-helps-manage-

stress-and-anxiety/#:~:text=Protein%20helps%20stabilize%20blood%20
sugar&text=With%20acute%20or%20short%2Dterm

25. Cherpak, C. E. (2019). Mindful Eating: A Review Of How The Stress-Digestion-Mindfulness Triad May Modulate And Improve Gastrointestinal And Digestive Function. *Integrative Medicine: A Clinician's Journal, 18*(4), 48–53. https://www.ncbi.nlm.nih.gov/pmc/articles/PMC7219460/#:~:text=Mindful%20eating%20is%20an%20opportunity

26. *2022's Ultimate list of quotes about sleep.* (2022, January 14). Bearaby. https://bearaby.com/blogs/the-lay-low/sleep-quotes

27. Vandergriendt, C. (2023, March 20). *How long can you go without sleep? Function, hallucination, more.* Healthline. https://www.healthline.com/health/healthy-sleep/how-long-can-you-go-without-sleep#:~:text=The%20longest%20recorded%20time%20without

28. Theobald, M., & Chai, C. (2022, August 9). *What happens when you don't sleep for days.* EverydayHealth.com. https://www.everydayhealth.com/conditions/what-happens-when-you-dont-sleep-days/#:~:text=At%2036%20Hours%3A%20Physical%20Health

29. Yurcaba, J. (2023, January 17). *Better sleep can improve stress response and increase positivity, study shows.* Verywell Mind. https://www.verywellmind.com/better-sleep-can-improve-stress-response-and-help-you-enjoy-positives-study-shows-5079820

30. *If you want to go fast go alone. If you want to go far go together. - African Proverb - Quotes Pedia.* (n.d.). Quotespedia. https://www.quotespedia.org/authors/a/african-proverbs/if-you-want-to-go-fast-go-alone-if-you-want-to-go-far-go-together-african-proverb/

31. *Manage stress: Strengthen your support network.* (2022, October 21). APA. https://www.apa.org/topics/stress/manage-social-support#:~:text=The%20benefits%20of%20social%20support

32. Touronis, V. (2022, April 1). *Social support and stress: how does it help?* My Online Therapy. https://myonlinetherapy.com/social-support-and-stress/#:~:text=A%202014%20study%20by%20the

33. Krowiak, S. (2020, March 11). *The vagus nerve: Your superhighway to physical, mental and emotional health.* Tune up Fitness. https://www.tuneupfitness.com/blog/vagus-nerve

34. Seladi-Schulman, J. (2023, February 14). *What is the vagus nerve?* Healthline. https://www.healthline.com/human-body-maps/vagus-nerve#problems

35. WomensMedia. (2021, April 15). *What the vagus nerve is and how to stimulate it for better mental Health.* Forbes. https://www.forbes.com/sites/womensmedia/2021/04/15/what-the-vagus-nerve-is-and-how-to-stimulate-it-for-better-mental-health/?sh=2140985e6250

36. *Why forest therapy can be good for your body and mind.* (n.d.). Health Essentials from Cleveland Clinic. https://health.clevelandclinic.org/why-forest-therapy-can-be-good-for-your-body-and-mind/

37. *Quotes about application of knowledge.* (n.d.). Quote Master. https://www.quotemaster.org/application+of+knowledge

38. *William Shakespeare Quote: "Give sorrow words; the grief that does not speak knits up the o-er wrought heart and bids it break."* (n.d.). Quotefancy. https://quotefancy.com/quote/7009/William-Shakespeare-Give-sorrow-words-the-grief-that-does-not-speak-knits-up-the-o-er

WORKBOOK 2

TOOLS TO REGULATE YOUR NERVOUS SYSTEM

Somatic, Cognitive & Lifestyle Techniques
To Create Calm, Relieve Stress & Reduce Anxiety

NOTES

NOTES

CHAPTER 1

Isn't it interesting that beneath our skin is the most complex organism on the planet. We own it. We use it. We rely on it for absolutely everything and yet we understand very little about it.

In this chapter, we got to see how amazing and intricate our central nervous system is.

Rather than just reading this, saying "wow" and then moving on, let's actually stop for a moment and embed a high-level understanding of how this system works.

You'll see a diagram below and you have the opportunity to label each of the major components of your nervous system.

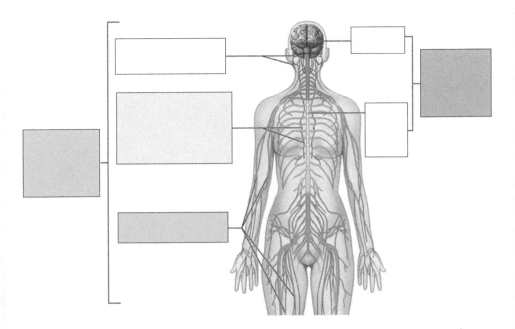

Spinal Nerves, Cranial Nerves, Brain, Spinal Cord, Autonomic Nervous System Ganglia, Central Nervous System, Peripheral Nervous System

REFLECTION JOURNAL:

In each chapter you'll have a chance to pause and reflect on what you've just discovered. This is a really important part of retaining more information. Plus, it's a nice break to reset, calm down and check in with yourself before you begin another chapter. In this moment of reflection, consider your own personal experiences and thoughts that relate to stress in your life. Write about your stress triggers, any coping mechanisms you've adopted (good and bad), and any patterns or insights you notice.

STRESS INVENTORY

Often we can become so used to the stress we experience that we have stopped recognizing it as stress. It's just become part of life. To calm our nervous system, we need to be aware of what is unsettling it. Take a moment to think about the stressors in your life. Below you'll see some common areas that are the cause of stress. You may likely have your own and there's room to add those too. Label each stressor and the impact it's having on your well-being. Becoming aware of these stressors will make the process of eliminating or reducing them actually possible.

Work

....

....

....

....

Colleagues

....

....

....

....

Family

....

....

....

....

Friends

....

....

....

....

Relationship

....

....

....

....

Health

....

....

....

Money

....

....

....

Other

....

....

....

....

....

....

....

CHAPTER 2

First, breathe ...

- In slowly while counting to four.

- Hold your breath for four counts before slowly releasing the air while counting to four.

- Repeat the cycle 10 times and feel your body is changing from being in a state of high stress to much calmer.

Well done. That's not hard to do but it's even easier not to do. I hope the exercise rewards you with a feeling of calm. I hope it settles your mind and body. I wish that you were frequently calm. I wish that this becomes a common state for you.

This chapter is particularly important. It establishes the premise of the book itself - the importance of balancing the PNS and SPNS. To secure your understanding of the points in this chapter, here is a short summary of what you've read:

1. The autonomic nervous system, particularly the sympathetic and parasympathetic divisions, plays a crucial role in the body's stress response and restoration of calm.

2. The sympathetic nervous system (SNS) activates during stress, leading to physical changes like increased heart rate, pupil dilation, and decreased digestion, while the parasympathetic nervous system (PSNS) restores calm by constricting pupils, slowing heart rate, and promoting circulation to vital systems.

3. In modern society, prolonged exposure to stressors can lead to imbalances between the SNS and PSNS, resulting in negative effects on physical and mental health.

4. Techniques such as massage, meditation, yoga, exercise, and adequate sleep can help activate the parasympathetic response, promoting relaxation and well-being.

5. Understanding and harnessing the mind-body connection empowers individuals to manage their stress response effectively, leading to improved overall wellness.

REFLECTION JOURNAL

Take time to digest the points from this chapter and make your notes below. Think about the state that you most frequently occupy. How calm are you? How often? Then, importantly, think and write about the activities that you conduct regularly that manually switch on your Parasympathetic Nervous System. Are there any? Do they happen frequently? If not, what are the challenges that are getting in the way? As we explore more of these sorts of activities in later chapters, you'll understand more about the benefits of implanting them in your life. So, if there are things getting in the way now, what do you need to do to make space for these new, healthy activities? For example, you may write something like – "It's time for a full screen detox. I'm banning my eyes from any screens after 7pm, every day"

....

....

....

....

....

....

....

....

....

....

....

....

....

....

Finished? Well done. I hope these reflections are helping to settle the information in your mind and make it part of your new awareness, your new life.

Now, breathe

- In slowly while counting to four.

- Hold your breath for four counts before slowly releasing the air while counting to four.

- Do it 10 times to get your body feeling calmer and lighter. Feel your body wanting to move and sway. Feel the rigidity of your body melt. This feeling is immensely healthy for your entire body. Sickness resides in rigid human forms. Healing happens in your fluidity and peace.

When you're ready, return to the book for the final part of Chapter 2.

CHAPTER 3

Many people will find their way to exploring nervous system regulation following exposure to trauma. Perhaps you've arrived here via that path. Perhaps, like many, you're not sure whether your experiences constitute as traumatic.

Whilst it's never the objective to relabel innocuous events as past trauma, it's always the objective to live a life free from unnecessary suffering. Such suffering occurs when events with traumatic impact go unaddressed. Let's take a moment to discover if any such events are part of your past. Take a moment now to reflect on your own experiences or knowledge related to trauma.

Firstly, here are some simple yes or no questions. Your answers here are not prescriptive but if the number of yes's far outweigh the no's, it could be an indication that trauma is indeed a feature of your past.

QUESTION	ANSWER	
Do you experience a constant state of heightened anxiety?	YES ☐	NO ☐
Are you often angry and can't identify why?	YES ☐	NO ☐
Do you frequently feel depressed?	YES ☐	NO ☐
Do you constantly seek perfection in the things you do?	YES ☐	NO ☐
Are your thoughts and dreams disrupted by distressing memories or obsessive thoughts?	YES ☐	NO ☐
Are you able to identify what caused you the hurt you're feeling?	YES ☐	NO ☐

OK, well your responses above are interesting. Here are a few broader questions that may help you articulate your past in terms that may help you embark on a path to healing, should that be necessary.

Do you think anything you have experienced or witnessed constitutes a form of trauma? If so, and just for the sake of identifying it, what were those events? You don't need to be elaborate in your description.

....

....

....

If so, how do you think that past trauma affects you?

....

....

....

....

....

In relation to those experiences, you may find yourself reliving moments from the past when things that occur in the present remind you of your past trauma, even things that bear no obvious connection to the past. Those things are known as 'triggers'. Can you identify any examples of triggers that push you outside your window of tolerance, leading to hyperarousal or hypo arousal states?

....

....

....

....

....

Do you think the described therapeutic approaches could be helpful in addressing your trauma and restoring a state of calm? If so, explain how below. Articulating this may be the thing that prompts you to take action rather than just thinking about it.

....

....

You've been given a short tour of the trauma therapy landscape. Rather than being told by others which form of therapy is right for you, with the information in this chapter, you're able to take an active role in deciding which mode of therapy you feel is most suitable.

There's a lot of information in the chapter and trying to remember it all will be very difficult so the table below is a place to keep notes on each form of therapy you learn about. You can also record contact details of therapists local to you. Plus you can keep notes on your experiences with any of these forms of therapy that you try.

COGNITIVE PROCESSING THERAPY

Notes - a summary of what it's about, its relevance to me, my general interest in it

My local therapist

My experience with it (post-treatment)

EMDR

Notes - a summary of what it's about, its relevance to me, my general interest in it

My local therapist

My experience with it (post-treatment)

PROLONGED EXPOSURE THERAPY

Notes - a summary of what it's about, its relevance to me, my general interest in it

My local therapist

My experience with it (post-treatment)

SOMATIC EXPERIENCING

Notes - a summary of what it's about, its relevance to me, my general interest in it

My local therapist

My experience with it (post-treatment)

TALK THERAPIES

Notes - a summary of what it's about, its relevance to me, my general interest in it

My local therapist

My experience with it (post-treatment)

MOVEMENT PRACTICE

Notes - a summary of what it's about, its relevance to me, my general interest in it

My local therapist

My experience with it (post-treatment)

CHAPTER 4

We've created a week of mindfulness and meditation practices for you below. And, as usual, there is space for you to reflect and complete your journal notes. Take a deep breath before you continue. Then write ...

REFLECTION JOURNAL

As you make your notes below, consider how this chapter was relevant to you. What difference would these practices make to you? How will you use this information to manage your own stress? Which of the practices will make their way into your life? How and when? What will you need to give up to make room for them? That could even include your attitude towards some of them ...

....

....

....

....

....

....

....

....

LearnWell, Tools To Regulate Your Nervous System WORKBOOK

HEALTH RECORD

From now on, you will see prompts to record your physical, mental, and emotional state each time you write. Observing the changes will provide evidence for the impact of your new thinking and practices and it will provide fuel for your ongoing maintenance of a healthier nervous system.

Physically, I am

....

....

Mentally, I feel

....

....

Emotionally, I am experiencing

....

....

A WEEK OF MINDFULNESS

We have created a schedule of mindfulness and meditation for you. Set time aside each day for a week and make these simple activities part of your life. They will genuinely make a difference.

DAY 1: MINDFUL BREATHING

☐ Find a quiet space and set a timer for 5 minutes.

☐ Sit comfortably and close your eyes.

☐ Take a few deep breaths, focusing on the sensation of the air entering and leaving your body.

☐ Shift your attention to your breath, noticing the rise and fall of your abdomen with each inhale and exhale.

☐ When your mind wanders, gently bring your focus back to your breath without judgment.

☐ Practice this mindful breathing exercise for the full 5 minutes.

DAY 2: MINDFUL WALKING

☐ Choose a peaceful outdoor location for a mindful walk.

☐ As you start walking, bring your attention to the sensation of your feet touching the ground.

☐ Notice the movement of your body, the sounds around you, and any smells or sights.

☐ If your mind starts to wander, gently guide your focus back to the present moment and your walking experience.

☐ Engage all your senses and stay fully present during the walk.

☐ Take at least 10 minutes for your mindful walk.

DAY 3: PROGRESSIVE MUSCLE RELAXATION

- ☐ Find a comfortable spot where you can lie down and relax.
- ☐ Start at your toes and gradually tense and release each muscle group in your body, working your way up to your head.
- ☐ As you tense each muscle group, hold the tension for a few seconds, and then release, allowing the muscles to relax fully.
- ☐ Focus on the sensations in each muscle group as you tense and release them.
- ☐ Take your time and move through all the major muscle groups in your body.
- ☐ Spend about 15-20 minutes practicing progressive muscle relaxation.

DAY 4: MINDFULNESS IN DAILY ACTIVITIES

- ☐ Throughout the day, choose a few routine activities to practice mindfulness.
- ☐ Whether it's brushing your teeth, eating a meal, or washing dishes, bring your full attention to the present moment.
- ☐ Notice the sensations, sounds, smells, and tastes associated with each activity.
- ☐ Avoid multitasking and be fully engaged in the task at hand.
- ☐ Whenever your mind starts to wander, gently bring it back to the activity you're performing.
- ☐ Aim to practice mindfulness in at least three different activities during the day.

DAY 5: LOVING-KINDNESS MEDITATION

- [ ] Find a quiet and comfortable space for your meditation practice.
- [ ] Begin by focusing on your breath for a few minutes to calm the mind.
- [ ] Then, bring to mind someone you care about and silently repeat phrases of loving-kindness towards them.
- [ ] Examples of phrases: "May you be happy. May you be healthy. May you be safe. May you live with ease."
- [ ] After a few minutes, extend these wishes to yourself, a neutral person, and even to someone you may have difficulty with.
- [ ] Stay with the practice for about 10-15 minutes, cultivating feelings of compassion and kindness.

DAY 6: BODY SCAN MEDITATION

- [ ] Lie down in a comfortable position and bring your attention to your body.
- [ ] Slowly scan through your body from head to toe, noticing any sensations or areas of tension.
- [ ] As you come across tension or discomfort, bring your awareness to those areas and consciously relax them.
- [ ] Take your time and be fully present in each part of your body as you scan through it.
- [ ] If your mind wanders, gently guide it back to the body scan.
- [ ] Practice the body scan meditation for about 20 minutes.

DAY 7: MINDFUL EATING

- [ ] Choose one meal or snack to practice mindful eating.
- [ ] Before you start, take a moment to appreciate the appearance, smell, and colors of your food.
- [ ] As you eat, savor each bite and pay attention to the flavors, textures, and sensations

CHAPTER 5

REFLECTION JOURNAL

Think about your current stress-to-exercise ratio. In chapter 1 you identified some of the stressors in your life. Those events that are causing you stress. How much balance do you create with exercise? For example, for every hour you spend in a stressful environment, how many minutes or hours are you counteracting that with exercise? What may need to change in your life to create a healthier balance? What will the challenges be that interfere with your ability to do this? How will you overcome them? Perhaps make some notes about where, when and with whom you'll be able to start some of these forms of exercise. For example, where is your local yoga studio? How can you attend a class? When in your day could you make time for a walk in nature? Where would you go?

....

....

....

....

....

....

....

....

LearnWell, Tools To Regulate Your Nervous System WORKBOOK

HEALTH RECORD

Get into the habit of checking in with yourself and becoming familiar with how you're feeling. Continue the habit below. Even if it's only been a day or so since you did it last time. Every day counts on your journey to peacefulness.

Physically, I am

....

....

Mentally, I feel

....

....

Emotionally, I am experiencing

....

....

CALENDAR OF CALM

Below you'll see a list of the exercises referred to in Chapter 4. You'll also see a calendar of 30 days. Choose those exercises you'd like to perform and place them on days throughout the calendar. Then make tomorrow Day 1 and begin!

Don't create a calendar that doesn't match reality at all. Create something that you genuinely believe you can achieve. At the end of each day, wherever you committed to and then completed the exercise, give yourself a point. If you get to 15 points by the end, you deserve a massage, a facial, a movie night or any other form of nervous system love!

You can use the letter abbreviations to indicate which exercise you are going to do on each day.

Y = Yoga

R = Resistance Training

A = Aerobic Exercises

B = Brisk Walking In Green Spaces

T = Engage in Team Sports

M = Mindful Movement Practices

E = Breathing Exercises

W = Walking Meditation

S = Stretching Exercises

F = Any Other Form of Exercise

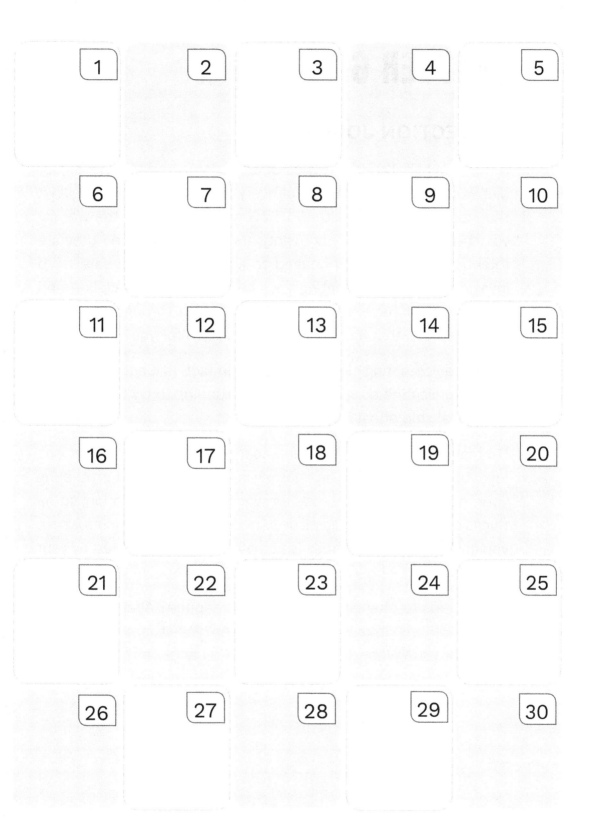

CHAPTER 6

REFLECTION JOURNAL

If we were to follow the advice of advertisers and the media, our diet would be a combination of every type of food that is against the interests of our health. So, how are you going in the war for your health? The enemy is mighty and they're loud and they are relentless? Have you managed to keep your castle safe from invasion? Are you protecting your health through discipline and education? Or have a few messages gotten through that have convinced you that alcohol and soda is good for you?

What are you eating? Is it helping? Or, in fact, is it actually part of a self-medicating program that you're running to try to keep your emotional ship afloat?

For many, this chapter will be an important revelation. That diet isn't just about losing weight and getting in shape. It's about protecting your mental health. For those for whom this *is* a revelation, some things may need to change. True? Are there areas of your life where you can see that your stress is actually being exacerbated by your diet?

What needs to change? When will that happen? Also write down the reason WHY that is going to happen? What is making this a MUST for you? What do you have to get a handle on?

....

....

....

....

....

....

....

HEALTH RECORD

Now with a little more time having past, how are you feeling?

Physically, I am

....

....

Mentally, I feel

....

....

Emotionally, I am experiencing

....

....

SHOPPING LIST

It's one thing to read about a great new diet. It's another thing entirely when you're staring at the grocery shelves wondering whether the book said walnuts or peanuts ...

So, to make it easier, we've created a shopping list for you that will fill your pantry with all the ingredients you'll need to nurture your nervous system. Below that we've even created a list of recipes that are all possible with the ingredients on the list.

Santé (to your health!)

PROTEINS	GRAINS	FRUITS	VEGETABLES	NUTS AND SEEDS	OTHER ITEMS
Chicken breast	Oatmeal	Berries (e.g., strawberries, blueberries, raspberries)	Broccoli	Almonds	Honey
Salmon	Quinoa		Asparagus	Walnuts	Dark chocolate (70% cocoa or higher)
Shrimp	Brown rice		Spinach	Pumpkin seeds	Kimchi (fermented vegetables)
Greek yogurt	Whole wheat couscous	Bananas	Cherry tomatoes	Chia seeds	Olive oil
			Cucumbers	Sesame seeds	Chamomile tea
					Milk

Remember to adjust the quantities based on your needs and preferences.

STRESS MANAGEMENT COOKING BOOK

We have created a simple collection of recipes that you will be able to make using the ingredients found on the grocery shopping list above (and some of the basics you'll have in your pantry already). Of course, not every recipe may suit your preference, but we're sure you'll find inspiration from some of them. Particularly the delicious desserts!

Breakfast

QUINOA PORRIDGE

INGREDIENTS:	Cooked quinoa, milk, honey, berries
INSTRUCTIONS:	Heat cooked quinoa with milk in a saucepan. Sweeten with honey and top with berries.

GREEK YOGURT PANCAKES

INGREDIENTS:	Greek yogurt, eggs, whole wheat flour, honey
INSTRUCTIONS:	Mix Greek yogurt, eggs, whole wheat flour, and honey to make a pancake batter. Cook pancakes on a griddle.

BERRY OATMEAL

INGREDIENTS:	Oatmeal, Greek yogurt, berries, honey
INSTRUCTIONS:	Cook oatmeal according to package instructions, top with Greek yogurt, fresh berries, and a drizzle of honey.

BANANA WALNUT SMOOTHIE

INGREDIENTS:	Banana, Greek yogurt, almond milk, walnuts, honey
INSTRUCTIONS:	Blend banana, Greek yogurt, almond milk, walnuts, and honey until smooth.

Snack

HUMMUS AND VEGGIE PLATTER

INGREDIENTS:	Hummus, carrot sticks, cucumber slices, bell pepper strips
INSTRUCTIONS:	Arrange carrot sticks, cucumber slices, and bell pepper strips on a platter. Serve with hummus for dipping.

YOGURT AND MIXED BERRY SMOOTHIE

INGREDIENTS:	Greek yogurt, mixed berries, almond milk, honey
INSTRUCTIONS:	Blend Greek yogurt, mixed berries, almond milk, and honey until smooth.

GREEK YOGURT PARFAIT

INGREDIENTS:	Greek yogurt, berries, honey, granola (optional)
INSTRUCTIONS:	Layer Greek yogurt, berries, honey, and granola (if desired) in a glass.

ALMOND BUTTER AND BANANA SLICES

INGREDIENTS:	Whole wheat toast, almond butter, banana
INSTRUCTIONS:	Spread almond butter on whole wheat toast and top with banana slices.

Lunch

GRILLED CHICKEN AND SPINACH SALAD

INGREDIENTS:	Grilled chicken breast, spinach, cherry tomatoes, cucumber, olive oil
INSTRUCTIONS:	Toss grilled chicken, spinach, cherry tomatoes, and cucumber in a bowl. Drizzle with olive oil as dressing.

SHRIMP QUINOA BOWL

INGREDIENTS:	Cooked quinoa, cooked shrimp, broccoli, cherry tomatoes, olive oil
INSTRUCTIONS:	Combine cooked quinoa, cooked shrimp, steamed broccoli, and cherry tomatoes in a bowl. Drizzle with olive oil.

SALMON SALAD WRAP

INGREDIENTS:	Cooked salmon, whole wheat wrap, spinach, cherry tomatoes, Greek yogurt
INSTRUCTIONS:	Fill a whole wheat wrap with cooked salmon, spinach, cherry tomatoes, and Greek yogurt as a dressing.

Dinner

BAKED SALMON WITH ASPARAGUS

INGREDIENTS: Salmon filet, asparagus, olive oil, lemon juice

INSTRUCTIONS: Place salmon filet and asparagus on a baking sheet. Drizzle with olive oil and lemon juice. Bake at 375°F (190°C) for 15-20 minutes.

CHICKEN STIR-FRY WITH BROWN RICE

INGREDIENTS: Chicken breast, mixed vegetables (e.g., broccoli, bell peppers), brown rice, soy sauce

INSTRUCTIONS: Stir-fry chicken breast and mixed vegetables in a pan. Serve over cooked brown rice. Add soy sauce for seasoning.

QUINOA-STUFFED ZUCCHINI BOATS

INGREDIENTS: Zucchini, cooked quinoa, black beans, diced tomatoes, shredded cheese

INSTRUCTIONS: Cut zucchini in half lengthwise and scoop out the center. Mix cooked quinoa, black beans, and diced tomatoes. Fill the zucchini boats with the mixture and sprinkle shredded cheese on top. Bake at 375°F (190°C) for 20-25 minutes.

TURKEY MEATBALLS WITH SPAGHETTI SQUASH

INGREDIENTS: Ground turkey, breadcrumbs, egg, garlic, spaghetti squash, marinara sauce

INSTRUCTIONS: Mix ground turkey, breadcrumbs, egg, and minced garlic to form meatballs. Bake meatballs in the oven. Meanwhile, cook spaghetti squash and heat marinara sauce. Serve the turkey meatballs over spaghetti squash with marinara sauce.

Dessert

BAKED APPLE WITH CINNAMON

INGREDIENTS: Apple, cinnamon, honey, walnuts (optional)

INSTRUCTIONS: Core the apple and place it in a baking dish. Sprinkle cinnamon and drizzle honey over the apple. Bake at 375°F (190°C) for 20-25 minutes. Top with crushed walnuts if desired.

BERRY YOGURT POPSICLES

INGREDIENTS: Greek yogurt, mixed berries, honey

INSTRUCTIONS: Blend Greek yogurt, mixed berries, and honey until smooth. Pour the mixture into popsicle molds and freeze until solid.

DARK CHOCOLATE COVERED STRAWBERRIES

INGREDIENTS: Dark chocolate, strawberries

INSTRUCTIONS: Melt dark chocolate, dip strawberries in the melted chocolate, and let them cool until the chocolate hardens.

GREEK YOGURT WITH HONEY AND WALNUTS

INGREDIENTS: Greek yogurt, honey, walnuts

INSTRUCTIONS: Serve Greek yogurt in a bowl, drizzle with honey, and top with crushed walnuts.

CHAPTER 7

Zzzzzzzzz ... oh, good morning. I must have slept in!

Where were we ... ? That's right - sleeping. So, how's yours?

Below you'll see a simple table that allows you to measure the quality of your sleep. It's repeated 3 times so you can revisit this to repeat the process at various intervals. You may like to do it:

- Now

- After you've upgraded your sleeping hygiene

- After an abnormal event in you life. Such as a high stress moment or a period of change.

The process is very simple. Just rate each sleep characteristic out of 10. It's subjective but if you repeat the process enough you'll establish some consistency in your criteria.

Score / 10		
	Satisfaction	How satisfied you are with the sleep you get.
	Alertness	Rate how alert and refreshed you feel during the day.
	Timing	The consistency in the times you go to bed and wake up.
	Efficiency	How much of the time you're in bed you sleep.
	Duration	This determines whether you've gotten enough sleep.
	AVERAGE	Add each score and divide the total by 5. This becomes your point of comparison for subsequent measures.

Score / 10		
	Satisfaction	How satisfied you are with the sleep you get.
	Alertness	Rate how alert and refreshed you feel during the day.
	Timing	The consistency in the times you go to bed and wake up.
	Efficiency	How much of the time you're in bed you sleep.
	Duration	This determines whether you've gotten enough sleep.
	AVERAGE	Add each score and divide the total by 5. This becomes your point of comparison for subsequent measures.

Score / 10		
	Satisfaction	How satisfied you are with the sleep you get.
	Alertness	Rate how alert and refreshed you feel during the day.
	Timing	The consistency in the times you go to bed and wake up.
	Efficiency	How much of the time you're in bed you sleep.
	Duration	This determines whether you've gotten enough sleep.
	AVERAGE	Add each score and divide the total by 5. This becomes your point of comparison for subsequent measures.

OK, with those results in mind, there's probably some room for improvement.

Here's the list of sleep hygiene practices referred to in the book, They are arranged in a table with some added features. The hygiene practice is shown next to a check box. Underneath that is space for you to make a note on what actions would be required for you to activate this sleep hygiene practice in your life.

Go ahead and run through the list. You don't have to do everything at once but let this serve as a reference whenever you feel like your sleep needs some upgrading. Based on the results above, perhaps that's now ... ??

☐ Define your sleep schedule by going to bed and waking up at roughly the same time every day.

```
.............................................................................
.............................................................................
.............................................................................
```

☐ Treat sleep like the priority it should be in your life. By this I mean avoid giving preference to having fun, screentime or working over sleeping.

```
.............................................................................
.............................................................................
.............................................................................
```

☐ Daytime naps can be fun and are a real treat, but sleeping during the day can affect your sleep at night and be the reason you're struggling to fall asleep. So, if you struggle to fall asleep, cut back on your daytime naps.

☐ When making changes to your sleep routine, do it gradually. Creating any sudden transitions in this regard can overthrow your entire sleeping routine.

☐ A night time routine indicates to your brain what is about to happen to help it prepare for sleep by slowing down. It also helps to go to bed every night at the same time.

☐ Step away from electronic devices for at least 30 minutes (preferably longer) before you want to sleep. The blue light of these devices keeps your brain active and will prevent sleep. Instead, grab a book and read to relax your mind.

☐ A warm shower or bath before bedtime can also help calm the mind and body.

☐ Refrain from making any mental connections linked to activity with your bedroom. It means that it is best to keep your bedroom for what it is intended, sleeping or as a place to relax. If you're in the habit of bringing work to bed, you're establishing a mental connection that your bedroom is a place of work instead of rest. Take it a step further and keep your phone out of the bedroom too. Or, at least, out of the bed.

....

....

....

☐ Bright light can also keep sleep at bay, so opt for dim light to create a relaxing environment.

....

....

....

☐ Some precautions you can take to support good sleep start during the day. Ensure enough exposure to sunlight, as this helps your circadian (sur-key-dee-uhn) rhythm. Circadian rhythm refers to the mental, physical, and behavioral changes within 24 hours. These changes are regulated by exposure to light and darkness.

....
....
....

☐ An increased activity level also contributes to nighttime exhaustion and will help you to sleep better.

....
....
....

☐ Reducing or eliminating smoking, a known cause of poor quality sleep, will be helpful.

....
....
....

☐ Late-night dining requires digestion when the body should be allocating resources to functions other than digestion.

☐ Alcohol may make you sleepy, but consuming alcoholic drinks close to bedtime will result in poor-quality sleep, keeping the body from entering a healthy sleeping cycle.

CHAPTER 8

You've felt it – the blissful joy of friends. An effortless conversation. Time that evaporates without your awareness. In those moments, stress melts, shoulders drop, and blood pressure plummets. They are beautiful moments. Poetic, even. Some may say they are what makes life worth living.

If you are at all inclined to agree then surely it makes sense to create more of them. Let's do that.

First, we need people. Who have you got? Who's in your support network? Who can you call for a laugh, a download, a cry, perhaps?

I know I have friends but I also know that I can easily let the distractions and urgency of work, family, and general life obscure my recollection of them. Yes, I forget who they are. I forget what they're up to. I forget to call them.

Years ago I realized that if I was ever going to be intentional about my relationships, I had to treat them with no less diligence than I was giving to other aspects of my life. I used to spend more time organizing my utility bills than my friends' contact details. I knew more about my colleagues' lives than my closest friends. That was not OK and in the very moment I had this thought, I took action. Not over-the-top, knee-jerk, manic action. Sensible, simple action. I just started with a list. I just sat and carefully thought about who my friends actually were.

Below here is something that replicates the list I made. And below that is an exercise that will hopefully form a habit that will inject energy, love and currency into your own relationships.

Let's start here. Write down all the people that you want to maintain contact with. Remember - that's not everyone. Some folks just don't support you and the your healthiest, stress-free self. Your list ought to include those that will offer authentic, helpful support. Not just people that will take your calls.

MY PEOPLE

MY PEOPLE

OK, here's now to maintain your network. Every day for 7 days, choose 5 names from the list above and make contact with each of the five people. For some it will be a text message. For others, a letter in the mail (!). And for others, an actual, old-school, in-person home drop-in!

Choose the 5 people, write down their names and following the interaction, make a quick note. For example: Sent text via Facebook saying hey.

Of course, initially, you'll take comfort in contacting the 'safe' people – your current friends and family. Later on, though, you'll start to stretch the boundaries. The people that will find their way onto your list will be those with whom you've got some repair work to do. You'll start to add people that you don't know well but with whom you wish to build a better relationship. This simple tool will be the pillar upon which your support network is built.

Please actually do this exercise. It will reveal 2 things - what a difference it makes when you show people you're thinking of them. That alone will reveal to you how important your role is in the lives of others. Also, for some people, it will actually reveal how little time you're currently investing in your relationships. Trust me, you do not want to wait for a time of crisis to be trying to revive relationships you've ignored.

Do this exercise strictly for 7 days in a row. If you do, there's a chance it will become a habit. If it becomes a habit and you maintain it for 6 months, your life will become FULL of amazing interactions. All of which will serve to significantly lower your stress … and theirs! Not to mention the social events you'll be part of, the friendships you'll reinforce, the family unity you'll foster and so many other beautiful things.

DAY 1	
Name	**Note**

DAY 2	
Name	**Note**

DAY 3

Name	Note

DAY 4

Name	Note

DAY 5	
Name	**Note**

DAY 6	
Name	**Note**

DAY 7	
Name	**Note**

CHAPTER 9

We discovered the hidden, often-unknown Vagus Nerve and the incredible measure of control this nerve has over so many bodily functions. To know it's power and not utilize it would be a travesty. So, we also shared several exercises designed to 'lift the vagal tone'. Or, to positively affect the vagus nerve.

You can see these activities listed below. They appear in the table and we'd love to see you at least try each one and make a decision on those you'll incorporate into your daily life. So, in the left hand column you can place a tick once you've completed the exercise and underneath there is space to keep your notes on the impact you experienced following the exercise. Your notes should be a reflection of your feelings, particularly as they relate to your perceived levels of stress and relaxation.

The notes on how to perform each exercise are shown below the table.

☐ Eye Movement Technique

☐ The Half Salamander Exercise

☐ Gargling, Singing, Humming, And Chanting

☐ Laughter. Not just accidental laughter but laughter you actively pursued or created

☐ Belly Breathing

☐ Stimulating The Diving Reflex

☐ [Your favourite way to relax] _____

[text box]

☐ Forest Bathing

[text box]

☐ Foot Rubs

[text box]

Eye Movement Technique

This is a great way to begin to activate the vagus nerve and improve its stimulation to regulate your stress response.

1. Get comfortable on your back with your hands behind your head.

2. Interweave your fingers.

3. Start by looking straight ahead of you at the ceiling above.

4. Without moving your head, look as far as possible to the right.

5. Hold this position until you spontaneously yawn or swallow.

6. Only then can you return to the starting position, looking straight ahead.

7. Repeat the exercise, looking to the other side until your body spontaneously yawns or swallows.

What has just happened? By moving your eyes in this manner, you actively connect the eight suboccipital (sub-oc-cip-i-tal) muscles with those responsible for moving your eyes. The suboccipital muscles are located in four groups at the back of your neck in the same area where your vagus nerve is connected and their proximity allows for potential interactions and influences between the two. This is one very simple way to activate the vagus nerve to establish a state of greater calm.

The Half Salamander Exercise

This exercise can be done seated, so you can activate it anywhere you find yourself needing to activate your vagus nerve to lower your stress levels. This exercise is highly effective in activating the vagus nerve. So, try it once you're comfortable with the previously mentioned technique.

1. Keep your head straight while looking to the right as far as possible.

2. Then tilt your head to the right toward your shoulder while maintaining your view.

3. Hold this position for a minute.

4. Bring back your eyes and head to the center, a neutral state ahead of you.

5. Look to the left while holding your head straight before tilting your head toward your left shoulder.

6. Hold this position again for a minute before returning to your neutral state, looking right ahead. As the vagus nerve plays a pivotal role in breathing, you can also use your body to activate the vagus nerve through breathing exercises.

The eye movements this activity is based upon have been linked to overall brain activation and positive effects on the autonomic nervous system. Tilting your head to the side while maintaining your gaze can stretch and engage the muscles and tissues in your neck and upper body. This movement can help release tension, promote blood flow, and influence the activity of nerves, including those connected to the vagus nerve.

Gargling, Singing, Humming, And Chanting

When you're ready to activate the benefits of these activities for yourself, find a quiet spot where you can chant the word *ohm* several times. Yes, this is the sound often associated with meditation or spiritual practice. It is said to have calming and centering effects on the mind and body, helping to induce a state of relaxation, focus, and spiritual connection.

Laughter

Laughter can lift your mood and boost your immune system so don't wait for it to happen. Go and make it happen. Spend time with people that you know will make you laugh. Watch funny films, go to the comedy. Laughter is your medicine so go get a hero's dose.

Belly Breathing

A technique where you deliberately breathe so deeply that your diaphragm moves up and down in conjunction with the chest cavity expansion. You can succeed with this breathing exercise in several ways, and while any version will do, I recommend the steps below.

1. Place one hand on your stomach and the other on your chest.

2. Take a deep breath and feel how your chest cavity expands, pushing your hand up before the diaphragm pushes your belly up to make room for your chest cavity to expand.

3. While taking these deep breaths, your heart rate slows, and your blood pressure drops simultaneously.

Other simple tricks are to make your exhales a bit longer than your inhales. By exhaling longer than you inhale, your body immediately shifts into a state of relaxation. Try it now. Inhale for four counts, hold your breath, and exhale for six counts. Repeat a few times and see how well it works.

Stimulating The Diving Reflex

Just splashing your face with cold water will activate the Diving Reflex. You can also rub an ice cube on your face for instant improvement. The cold exposure will immediately slow your heart rate, relax your body, and cause your anxiety to plummet.

Foot Rubs

Whether it's a foot rub, a sauna or a night at a comedy show, lifting your vagal tone should be the intention behind as many daily activities as possible. Find the activities that you love and have immediate access to and make them part of your regular routine.

Forest Bathing

Spend time in green spaces, like a forest, and to shift your focus to the sights, sounds, and scents surrounding you. The technique forces you into a greater state of mindfulness. By getting swept away by your surroundings, you enjoy an emotional calm, forcing your brain to stop ruminating, worrying, or anticipating what will happen next.

CHAPTER 10

We're going to build a plan now. A plan that will incorporate much of what you've read and learned. This plan will help you to manage your stress, increase your calm and invoke a sense of peace. It uses 4 steps, as follows:

Step 1: Identify The Problem You're Facing

This step involves a moment, or several moments, of truth. Where you give up the act, let down your guard and let the truth of your circumstances prevail.

Where are you experiencing stress? Your immediate response might be to dismiss the question. You may have become so used to the stress that it's no longer stress, it's just life. You may have built up such a tolerance to the pressure you're facing that you've stopped hoping it would cease.

If someone else stepped into your shoes for a day, how would they feel? What challenges would they find stressful? What would they struggle to cope with?

As you adopt their point of view, make a list of your stressors.

Here are some common ones that may prompt your thinking. But don't stop at headlines. Get into the detail. It's not just work, it's that jerk Lisa who constantly interrupts me with her stupid questions and gossip all day. It's the unpaid electricity bill that means I'm getting calls from the power company after hours. It's the fact that I'm trying to fall pregnant and it feels like it's never going to happen for me.

Once you've reviewed the list below and given your own circumstances proper thought, make a list in the space of your stressors below:

- Health concerns

- The state of your relationships

- Financial stress

- Life changes

- Emotional problems

Personal beliefs can trigger stress. Some examples of such beliefs are beliefs related to religion, politics, or beliefs linked to your value system. The latter occurs when your values conflict with the views of others or those in your environment.

When you're discriminated against or even just witnessing discrimination.

Environmental factors, like disasters, poverty, or oppression.

Your career can trigger stress in several ways.

....

....

....

....

....

....

....

It's impossible to live a life without stress. However, it's entirely possible for you to reduce the frequency with which stress interrupts your life. You can put yourself in different situations, spend time with different people, stop talking about stressful things, with people who seem to get a kick out of winding you up.

What others do is not your responsibility. What you do is. So, what can you do to minimize your exposure to the stressors you've listed above. For example, can you leave home an hour earlier so you're stuck in traffic for so long? Can you wear earplugs at night to prevent the neighbors from disrupting your sleep? Can you tell your boss the truth about your workload and your overwhelm at the responsibility you've been given?

If there's a stressor in your life that is causing your nervous system to become disregulated and it's possible for you to eliminate the source of stress but, for whatever reason, you decide not to, that stress is now your fault, regardless of who is causing the stress.

So, now's the time to take responsibility for your peace and calm. Let's eliminate all unnecessary stress. On the lines below, write down a plan for how you'll attack your list of stressors. Get creative, get ruthless, get aggressive if that's going to help. Just make sure that you prioritize peace and health over any short-term, uncomfortable conflict.

....

....

....

....

....

....

....

....

....

....

....

....

....

Step 2: Taking Care Of Your "Vehicle"

Now you've got a list of the things in your life that are increasing your stress and, hopefully, a brilliant game plan for how to eliminate as many of them as possible. However, we all know that we can't and, frankly, don't want to get rid of *all* our stress. Some stress is helpful. It let's us know when things are important. Stress that persists indefinitely is not good. Stress as a signal to the priorities in our lives can be good. So, some stress will always exist. As a consequence, we need ways to manage the stress that occurs.

So, you've read the book, you're discovered the tools, you know that there are ways to live well in peace, despite stress. The question is – which tools are you going to use, when and with what level of frequency.

It's commitment time. Not to me. Not to anyone else. Just to yourself. Now it's time to put pen to paper and decide what you'll commit to for the sake of your own good health.

Reflect on what you've read. Go back through the notes you've made in this Workbook. Skim through the book again and remind yourself of what's available. Then, write your plan.

What appears below will be those things you are committing to. Go!

Step 3: Address Your Emotions

Could you describe your current emotional state? If you have never had to or even wanted to articulate how you feel, your emotions remain largely unknown. It's hard for you to understand what's happening and almost impossible for anyone to help you make sense of what you're experiencing. You create an extra, unnecessary burden for yourself by just putting up with the emotions that arrive instead of acknowledging them, describing them, perhaps sharing them with others and actively seeking a resolution to the ones that don't serve. Shakespeare said "Give sorrow words; the grief that does not speak knits up the o-er wrought heart and bids it break."[37.] I think what he means is "Express your sorrow through words; if your grief remains unspoken, it tightens your burdened heart and eventually causes it to break."

Below is an opportunity to express yourself in writing. It can remain strictly private if you choose but you may decide to share it those in your support network (Chapter 8). You may even take these words to your spiritual practice and pray over them. These expressions may form the basis of your meditation, mindful movement, breathing exercises, or other techniques we've discussed.

I know you'll find this a powerful exercise, particularly if you're not in the habit of sharing your thoughts or emotions freely.

So, if you're being honest, how do you *really* feel?

....

....

....

....

....

....

....

....

....

....

....

....

....

....

....

Good on you. That's brave. That's also the product of the life you're living – the stress, the joy, the wins, losses and the mental patterns you've developed to deal with it all. Is that how you want to feel? If so, great. Carry on. If there are parts that you're not satisfied with, now you know what to work on. Now you have something to potentially share with others –a therapist, friend, men's group, online support forum. If there's something to improve, you've taken a huge step towards finding the required solution. Now it's known. It's been described. It's real.

Well done.

Step 4: Give

What you gain from giving is an emotional surge equalled by few other actions. It could be your time or service, your money, your possessions or anything of value. Giving brings a sense purpose, pleasure, value, gratitude, belonging and accomplishment. Can you volunteer? Can you offer your services and contribute to the life of another? Can you offer your experience and advice on a topic or a cause? Can you help your neighbor? Can you take the clothes you no longer wear to the local thrift store? Can you join a movement, help a cause or even start one yourself?

 "You can never go broke giving money away"
J. Paul Getty.

If you're seeking a circuit-breaking stress relief, give. Put yourself in the way of people who need help. You'll quickly discover two things: (1) Your own value to others; and (2) the relative insignificance of your own problems.

What could you do? What are you willing to do? Use the space below to brainstorm the plan for your contributions. It will be perhaps the most satisfying, stress-neutralizing thing you'll do.

....

....

....

....

....

....

....

....

....

....

....

....

....

....

....

....

....

The four steps that you've just breathed your own life into form the basis of your nervous system regulation plan. Good work. I trust this will deliver significant benefits to you.

Made in the USA
Monee, IL
09 August 2024

63594355R00201